Balancing on Quicksand

"This book reads like the kind of writing we all want, really - an intimate conversation, riveting, unruly, a private 'in' to other worlds of feeling, without instruction or the impositions of academia, a broader canvas, open and porous, gently meandering through art, fiction, memoir and therapy. 'Balancing on Quicksand' is an inclusive act, (continuing to) disrupt the personal/professional boundary and psy-orthodoxies – the personal is (still) political, the political is (still) personal. Expect tears!"
—Professor Isabel Henton, *Regent's University London*

"Prof. Milton and his colleagues offer us a deeply engaging, stimulating and thought-provoking collection of reflective essays that eloquently illustrate the value and significance of relational thinking towards attaining psychological and social health and social justice. Each contributor's personal reflective journey of engaging with a key human dilemma in relation to power, politics and the relational is an invitation to the reader to reflect on our own stance and engagement with the key human dilemmas explored in this book."
—Dr. Stelios Gkouskos, *Roehampton University, London*

"Sometimes the release of a book comes at just the right time ... after a year of social distancing and COVID quarantine, I can think of no better time to read about how relational thinking plays out in the real lives and lived experiences of practicing psychotherapists as they grapple with the professional, personal, psychosocial, and political."
—Dr. Markus Bidell, *Hunter College, City University of New York*

Martin Milton
Editor

Balancing on Quicksand

Reflections on Power, Politics and the Relational

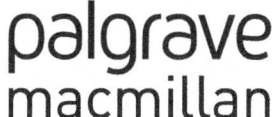

Editor
Martin Milton
Regent's University London
London, UK

ISBN 978-3-030-79135-3   ISBN 978-3-030-79136-0 (eBook)
https://doi.org/10.1007/978-3-030-79136-0

© The Editor(s) (if applicable) and The Author(s), under exclusive license to Springer Nature Switzerland AG 2021
This work is subject to copyright. All rights are solely and exclusively licensed by the Publisher, whether the whole or part of the material is concerned, specifically the rights of translation, reprinting, reuse of illustrations, recitation, broadcasting, reproduction on microfilms or in any other physical way, and transmission or information storage and retrieval, electronic adaptation, computer software, or by similar or dissimilar methodology now known or hereafter developed.
The use of general descriptive names, registered names, trademarks, service marks, etc. in this publication does not imply, even in the absence of a specific statement, that such names are exempt from the relevant protective laws and regulations and therefore free for general use.
The publisher, the authors and the editors are safe to assume that the advice and information in this book are believed to be true and accurate at the date of publication. Neither the publisher nor the authors or the editors give a warranty, expressed or implied, with respect to the material contained herein or for any errors or omissions that may have been made. The publisher remains neutral with regard to jurisdictional claims in published maps and institutional affiliations.

This Palgrave Macmillan imprint is published by the registered company Springer Nature Switzerland AG
The registered company address is: Gewerbestrasse 11, 6330 Cham, Switzerland

To those that have explored these paths and in whose tracks we follow. For those who will push further and extend our understandings and our treatment of our co-existents.

To Stuart, Harry and Jessie. As always, balancing me through the process.

Acknowledgements

I want to acknowledge the enthusiasm, courage and intrepidness of the contributors to this collection. None of the topics explored are necessarily easy to put into words, yet these authors managed superbly—and they did this without turning to the formulaic strategies that are so often utilised. They trusted a more creative process, one which led to more thoughtful essays and stories, that cross boundaries of professional, academic, creative and memoir writing. They trusted their ability to write, receive feedback and change direction as and when it proved imaginatively imperative. I am grateful for their resilience and the trust they placed in me.

I particularly appreciate the generosity to Dr. Hadjiosif for allowing me to utilise the heading of his chapter for the collection as a whole. As readers will imagine, settling on a title is not always easy, especially when there is an attempt to ensure that potential readers have a sense of what they are being invited to immerse themselves in. A book such as this, that explores diverse awkward, difficult and felt phenomena, was always going to be hard to title. In fact several provisional titles turned into mini-essays themselves. Miltos' title captures something of what each of the contributors is describing, they are all navigating difficult terrain, sometimes balancing on quicksand as they explore emotion in therapy, judgement and its uses, relationships—to authority, to animals or to art and more. So thank you Miltos.

Martin Milton

Contents

Introduction 1
Martin Milton

What Place Authority?

Rolling in the Muck, Dancing with the Law: A Story of "Addiction" and the Remaking of a Self 13
J. P. Marshall

Breaking the Rules 25
Alison Greenwood

Disturbing the Peace: Madame X vs Westminster Council 37
Martin Milton

The Reach of Reductionism

"Objective"-ication: Problems with Treating Judgement as Fact 49
Helen Damon

Animals: Aren't They Great? *Dale Judd*	59
Balancing on Quicksand: Making Sense of What "The Personal is Political" Means *Miltos Hadjiosif*	77

Judgement, Discrimination and Stigma

Drama of Phantom Hatred *Parizad Bathai*	97
Reflections from a Junkyard Room *Yetunde Ade-Serrano*	103
"I'm Not as Bad as You" *Carter Jacobs*	115
Is There Something You Need to Tell Us? *Julia Brewer*	125

The Uncanny

Being a Refugee in a World Without Refuge *Anastasios Gaitanidis*	139
An Uncanny Resemblance *Elena Manafi*	145
Making the Invisible Visible *Martin Milton*	155
And Finally …	163
Index	165

Notes on Contributors

Dr. Yetunde Ade-Serrano is a Chartered Psychologist and a Registered Practitioner Counselling Psychologist. She primarily works in Independent Practice. Her expertise focuses on race, culture and difference and promotes awareness of discrimination and discriminatory practices. Within this context, Yetunde is involved with teaching, research, providing clinical supervision, mentoring and examining doctoral theses within Counselling Psychology. She is the founder of the Black and Asian Counselling Psychologists' Group, a group that creates space for the voices and experiences of Counselling Psychologists from Black and Asian communities.

Ms. Parizad Bathai draws on her experience of being part of the Iranian diaspora to draw attention to the emotions embedded in migration, the western gaze and the longevity of racial and other assumptions. Pari worked as a counsellor/psychotherapist with refugees and asylum seeker for many years before moving to NHS primary and secondary care. Pari has since retired.

Dr. Julia Brewer is a Counselling Psychologist and trans and non-binary ally. If she's not working in her psychotherapy practice or running after small children,[1] she would hope to be reading, walking in the countryside or planning a travel adventure, but in reality, she is probably taking the opportunity to catch up on "Ru Paul's Drag Race".

Dr. Helen Damon is a Counselling Psychologist, Play Therapist, Filial Therapist and fellow of the Higher Education Academy (FHEA). She is a Lecturer, and Placement Coordinator, on the DPsych. Counselling Psychology at Regent's University London, and she sees clients for psychological therapy in private practice.

Dr. Anastasios Gaitanidis is a Relational Psychoanalytic Psychotherapist, Author, Editor and Supervisor. In addition to his clinical work as a psychoanalytic therapist, Anastasios has held appointments at Regent's University London and University of Roehampton. He is the Theory Editor of the *European Journal of Psychotherapy and Counselling* (EJPC) and an author of a substantial body of academic work including journal articles and edited books. His most recent book is entitled *The Sublime in Everyday Life: Psychoanalytic and Aesthetic Perspectives*.

Dr. Alison Greenwood is a Chartered Counselling Psychologist and has been incorporating ecotherapy practices in her work with clients for many years. In 2018, she left the NHS to set up the mental health charity, Dose of Nature (www.doseofnature.org.uk), and in collaboration with academics, clinicians and clients, she developed a ten-week "nature prescription" that has been embraced by GPs and other mental health practitioners as an effective and genuine alternative to medication and more traditional psychological interventions.

Dr. Miltos Hadjiosif is Senior Lecturer in Counselling Psychology at UWE Bristol. His scholarly work and clinical practice sit at the intersection of community psychology and psychotherapy. Miltos is a Committee Member of the BPS Community Psychology Section and has been involved with the organisation of the *Community Psychology Festival*

---

[1] Her own.

since its inception. He is passionate about decolonising psychology and addressing the privileging of intellect over affect in critical pedagogy.

Carter Jacobs[2] draws on his experiences of coming out, the HIV epidemic and the need for activism in much of his work. He sees activism as just another human and professional responsibility rooted in relationship and a way to navigate the power structures that exist everywhere we turn.

Dr. Dale Judd is a Chartered Counselling Psychologist and has long critiqued the psychological and psychotherapy professions. In this collection, he turns his attention to the way in which we selectively interpret our relationship with animals. He is a long-time supporter of animal welfare—particularly The League Against Cruel Sports, Four Paws International and Wood Green Animals Shelter in Cambridgeshire, from where he and his wife rehomed their pet cat, Noodles.

Dr. Elena Manafi continues to be a Counselling Psychologist and Existential Psychotherapist in private practice. Her passion for contradictions, paradoxes, existential philosophy and psychoanalysis continues to inform her clinical work as well as academic and research interests. She currently holds a senior lectureship at City University where she teaches for the Professional Doctorate in Counselling Psychology. During the pandemic, Elena took on running as an act of defiance; to her surprise she ended up enjoying it and intends to commit to the act.

Dr. J. P. Marshall awaiting registration as a Counselling Psychologist, continues to grapple with authority, including his own. He is presently attentive to the overshadowing, toe-treading (shredding?) nature of dominant narratives in the sense-making of many who "dance" with "mental health services", and would like to voice his love, here, for Ella and Rosa. J. P. is an activist, supporter of Black Lives Matter and Extinction Rebellion, and an advocate of sustained nonviolent direct action. He hopes to dance with you on the streets, soon. He will try not to tread on (or shred) your toes.

---

[2] This contributor uses a nom de plume/pseudonym.

Prof. Martin Milton, CPsychol, FBPsS, UKCP Reg is a Fellow of the British Psychological Society and Professor of Counselling Psychology at the School of Psychotherapy and Psychology at Regents University London. He also runs an independent practice in psychotherapy and supervision. Martin's research and teaching interests are related to the way that differences are constructed and experienced and the impact this has on us. Martin is an avid photographer and nature lover and has his photographs published in both photography and psychology publications.

Introduction

Martin Milton

We didn't need the coronavirus pandemic to remind us that we live in a complicated world, with diverse constituencies and ever-changing perspectives, but the pandemic has brought this complexity and all its problems into sharp relief. Again. The pandemic sits alongside other urgent issues, such as economic inequity, climate change, white supremacy, misogyny and homophobia. They all remind us that, whether we experience it individually or collectively, we are perpetually trying to balance on quicksand.

Quicksand—That takes me back. No matter how problematic we might assess Tarzan movies to be nowadays, I remember watching them avidly as a kid—my love of nature, and my desire to live with animals was extreme. But as well as all the wonderful possibilities these films evoked, I was terrified by the scenes of people walking into quicksand, that benign looking substance hidden by leaf fall, just waiting to suck

M. Milton (✉)
Regent's University London, London, UK
e-mail: miltonm@regents.ac.uk

© The Author(s), under exclusive license to Springer Nature Switzerland AG 2021
M. Milton (ed.), *Balancing on Quicksand*,
https://doi.org/10.1007/978-3-030-79136-0_1

people down, slowly, into a blind, suffocating nightmare. I remember desperately noting that one mustn't panic, one should never struggle, and you definitely shouldn't rush. It didn't matter that the closest quicksand to me was a couple of continents away, I absorbed the lessons that could save my life. Stay calm. Scour your surroundings and assess the area, spread yourself out atop the quicksand, breathe slowly, and make thoughtful, considered movements.

I have never had to extricate myself from *actual* quicksand, but I have found myself in many a sticky situation, where panic has not been helpful, nor has simply trying to bulldoze my way through life's dilemmas.

To navigate the quicksand of relationships and life's uncertainties—we have to balance the competing demands of instinct and intellect, being an individual and a part of groups, some that we fit into and some we are rejected from. We have to consider power too—our own, that of the Other and power that is woven into the systems we inhabit. This complexity can fascinate us, as is evidenced by the human preoccupation with the fields of sociology and psychology, our love of theatre, literature, and science and religion. But the complexity also scares, worries and confounds us too. These experiences often result in us trying to limit uncertainty and to "know" our world, concretely and absolutely. To make it—and the others it contains—conform to our wishes. So, for much of the time we follow history and habit, travelling the paths that others have trodden before us. "If it ain't broke, don't fix it" we say; "Why reinvent the wheel?" we ask. And for much of the time this strategy works. As a species we have colonised the entire planet and done so very effectively. There is clearly an advantage to this ability, we build on what is known and stand on the shoulders of giants.

All good. Right?

Maybe.

Maybe not?

Quick, rash and habitual decisions can also overlook nuance and complexity and can send you downwards into a pit of quicksand before you can shout "TARZAN!"

Our reliance on binary ways of knowing—and relating—can be unhelpful too. Not everything fits into an "either-or" way of seeing the world. Binary perspectives feed hierarchical understandings which, in turn, underpin assumptions that some are more worthy than others; the in-group is viewed as safe, the out-group as *inevitably* dangerous. These views often underpin discrimination and lead to inequality that benefits only those with access to power and resources, while severely disadvantaging those without. The more these views are accepted/experienced as truths, the less attuned we are to the subtle realities of life. We can feel less competent to deal with the wonderful messy, complicated, contrary aspects of experience. And this grasp for certainty isn't just for us as individuals, it guides policy and practice and risks maintaining ill-attuned relationships and the damage that these bring.

"Ill-attuned relationships"—the formality of discourse can make it sound relatively benign. And on occasion maybe it is. Some interpersonal blunders are relatively minor, yet we also see them form the basis of damaging policy. It is bad enough when this occurs *without* us thinking but it is worrying when we see policy and practice adopted as a deliberate strategy to exploit some and benefit others. In those circumstances, "ill-attuned relationships" may mean overt violent or exploitative relationships or it might refer to those structures that create inequality. Ill-attuned relationships come to be perceived as "normal" so they are hard to see, to challenge or to change.

This is part of a practice of "Othering", which contributors refer to. Othering exacerbates the tendency to view the world through the prism of "us and them" and to use power accordingly. A mistrust of "them" is behind much bullying and facilitates hate speech. Othering is there systemically—it underpinned (and continues to underpin) homophobic responses to the HIV/AIDS pandemic; Splitting and Othering is used as justification for political and religious colonialism; it manifests itself in bricks and mortar when disability is overlooked. The exploiting of binary thinking is also evident in the deliberate and wilful misrepresentation of the needs of minorities. It is hard to be racist, transphobic, misogynistic or to abuse the class system unless you are adept at splitting groups into "us and them".

The binary perspective isn't our only way of seeing things of course. It never has been—it is just utilised deliberately in the exercise of power. Sadly, minority groups are used to the fact that systems often leave it up to "them" to vocalise the need for greater attunement; women lead the challenge to misogyny; LGBTQ+ folk rail against trans-, bi- and homophobia; and disabled people remind others that much of the world is set up inappropriately. It is an artefact of power that the work to dismantle the unequal structures is left to those with less power and it requires investment in collaborative, relational ways of thinking and acting.

One way this is undertaken is through attention to, and expression of, the subjective. The objective cannot capture reality on its own, the personal aspects of experience are crucial. Attention to the personal, political and relational heighten awareness, offer hope that good communication, the breaking down of distance and mystery, can mean we are not doomed to a permanent state of ill-attuned relationships. We are offered new perspectives, we can be empathic and see things from another's eye. But only if it occurs to us to do so. Allport and Kramer were on to something when they developed their "Contact Hypothesis[1]".

Although our contemporary digitised, corporatised and economised worldviews obfuscate the fact, more relational, personalised ways of understanding have stood us in good stead over millennia and continue to do so. Although, of course, we put our own spin on it. We may, as Yetunde Ade-Serrano points out in her chapter, no longer have the opportunity to sit with village elders if we live in metropolitan London, but we find other ways to talk—on planes and trains, in classrooms and in pubs. Humans exist through "talk" of one form or another—we chat, we gossip, we text and we slide into people's DMs. On a bigger scale, media companies fund radio station phone-ins and despite the attack on psychotherapy this last few decades, people invest in their mental health and personal development by utilising insight oriented, relational forms of therapy. An array of professions utilise more relational approaches too—we see this under the guise of reflective practice in nursing, the applied psychologies, psychoanalysis and medicine. Professional practice is poor if it pays no attention to the attunement between practitioner and client, researcher and participant, policy maker and citizen. The personal and subjective experience is being reclaimed and rehabilitated.

---

[1] Allport and Kramer (1946).

This isn't a book about reflective practice per se. Rather, this book extends the idea to a wider array of situations people have to navigate. It shows that reflection and reflexivity are important when navigating the dilemmas that pervade our existence, and our relationships with others. Relational thinking allows us to understand how emotion, behaviour and individual investment all inform, colour and impact what we do. Being mindful of this helps us consider *why* we do what we do in the roles we inhabit, what the function of belief, of feeling and of action is, and the gains we hope to make.

The Book

Contributors to this book adopt reflective stances to engage with some of life's tricky and confusing moments. They explore diverse experiences, all of which have the potential to unsettle us, leave us feeling we are precariously balanced on quicksand. These are situations where to move too fast lands us in trouble, move too slowly and we sink. Contributors explore key human dilemmas in four broad areas—in relation to boundaries and authority, our reductionistic approaches to life, the damage done by judgement and discrimination and the very personal, and uncomfortable, experiences of the uncanny. While these *might* be seen as distinct areas, as readers will recognise from the critique above, they should *not* be thought of as mutually exclusive silos. They can't be. This conceptualisation is simply a loose framework to orientate the reader.

Within all of these areas, contributors go beyond the usual, formulaic academic script. Some are primarily emotional, some more socio-political and many very personal. Regardless of their focus, all of the contributors rise to the challenge of being reflective in their exploration of their chosen topic. Through these explorations, readers are offered examples of how useful a reflective stance can be, to understand some of the more meaningful things in life, or as a corrective to some of our power based, normative, instructive discourses. Contributions are as much "reflective analyses" as "academic scholar" outputs … although, once again, most of us would argue that this binary is neither fixed nor fully accurate.

Contributors privilege critical thinking and debate, they build upon what being-with-others has taught them.

In all of the chapters, readers are invited to take a moment, explore different arenas in which people report unsettled, uncertain and precarious aspects of life. This offers the reader a chance to be moved by the experience of another, to see dilemmas and complications anew. Yes, contributors see the world through their own lenses, but they also demonstrate ways in which we might be open to the new, or the different. They encourage us to absorb complexity, to think about it in varied and creative ways and reflect upon our own positions.

Contributors such as Carter Jacobs, Parizad Bathai and Anastasios Gaitanidis unpack some intimately personal experiences and reflect what can be learnt from them. Others, Elena Manafi, Helen Damon and Alison Greenwood included, reflect on encounters they have had in their professional roles and what they learnt. This does not mean that the reader must learn the same lesson. On the contrary, the book focusses on the "lessons we've learnt" rather than on an attempt at "expert instruction in the art of therapy, teaching or other professional tasks". This approach allows—possibly ***requires***—the reader to think, to respond and maybe to argue as they engage with the ideas expressed. This is why the contributors were asked to eschew any attempt to foreground "practitioner points" as some journals are so fond of doing. We all recognise that it is only by actively grappling with these issues, in a live manner, that there is any possibility of learning.

We all hope that chapters will function as a trigger to a curious and imaginative engagement with issues and that some readers will find the insights useful, others will find them the springboard to other, different ideas that the contributors maybe didn't consider. And that would be good.

Very good.

That is what this book aims to do.

Reference

Allport, G. W., & Kramer, B. M. (1946). Some roots of prejudice. *The Journal of Psychology, 22*(1), 9–39.

What Place Authority?

Power, authority and the policing of rules are ubiquitous aspects of human interaction and frequently part of what makes life so uncertain and precarious. Trying to identify useful, safe and ethical ways of being is hard, there is seldom one rule that suits all circumstances. Even as certain diktats suit some, maybe even a majority, they can still put others at a disadvantage, leaving at least some of us unsatisfied, ostracised or even criminalised. And as we have seen again only too clearly in recent years, power can be exercised with considerable malintent, silencing or erasing people and events.

The three chapters in this first part all encourage us to think about power, about ethics and about resistance, to think critically, enthusiastically and regularly. To consider our own relationships to power, and to the Other and the rules that are generated too. Without such a mindful engagement, a thoughtless "every man for himself" mentality (so tempting at times of struggle and limited resources) is all but guaranteed to lead to relational and social breakdown. Such a strategy tends to lead to those with power consolidating it and normalising policies and practices that are unfair, discriminatory and oppressive for the Other. And then what do we do? What do the disempowered do?

Often times the rules of resistance, the question of how to question or challenge inequality, suits the powerful more than the disempowered. Want to raise an issue? Email your MP, write them a letter or send a tweet we are told. Does this get a quick and effective response? Very often not. The same way we recognise that "well-mannered women rarely make history",[1] neither do any well-mannered minority. Not because of a lack of ability, but because power is used to write history as the powerful perceive it. In the meantime, the disempowered sink ever deeper into the quicksand. So other forms of resistance, one's deemed unsporting or illegal by the rule-writers, are sometimes used. And it is to this that these three contributions turn, exploring the meaning of boundaries, rules and rule-breaking.

J. P. Marshall takes a biographical approach to explore authority, resistance to certain forms of it and the ways in which people suffer if authority is exercised unthinkingly, without considering the meaning it has for people. Drug-taking, gang-life, violence and the place of prisons all feature in this account. JP's exquisitely intimate—and courageous—account is a wonderful example of the ways in which we can see the personal and the political being intertwined, the usefulness of recognising this but also the difficult work it entails. In this chapter JP notes the reductive aspect of diagnosis and problems associated with it.

Alison Greenwood utilises the lens of her profession to explore the notion of rules and rule-breaking as well. As a psychologist, Alison is attuned to the ways in which she, her clients, work contexts and the courts all wield power (to varying degrees), and sometimes in ways that appear confusing, contradictory and damaging. As Alison explores this, readers are invited to think "what would I do in this circumstance?" "To what degree am I sure about that?" And "if I am sure (we are certain many will not be) *why* am I so sure?" Alison's reflections also bring home questions as to when it is important, an ethical requirement even, to sometimes break rules.

In the final chapter, I explore the ways in which power and authority are often delegated to people who may not have the freedom to choose

---

[1] Uhlrich (1976).

how to exercise it, nor to use discretion in its application. The collision between Madame X and Westminster Council gives us a chance to consider the fact that sometimes, *Artists are here to disturb the peace. Otherwise, chaos'*.² Sometimes it is only through a thoughtful and creative engagement with power that a bridge can be found between the theoreticolegal and emotional dimensions of life. It may be that art is both resistance and unification in those circumstances.

References

Literary Conversations Series. (Undated). *Conversations with James Baldwin.* University Press of Mississippi.

Ulrich, L. T. (1976). *Vertuous women found: New England ministerial literature, 1668–1735* (p. 20). John Hopkins University Press.

---

² Literary Conversation Series.

Rolling in the Muck, Dancing with the Law: A Story of "Addiction" and the Remaking of a Self

J. P. Marshall

"To the [Law] thou art a check. When his foot is on the neck[1] *"*

"Chronic remorse, as all the moralists are agreed, is a most undesirable sentiment. If you have behaved badly, repent, make what amends you can and address yourself to the task of behaving better next time. On no account brood over your wrongdoing. Rolling in the muck is not the best way of getting clean.[2] *"*

I spent the first decade of my existence in the small working class and mostly white Catholic mining town of Birtley in north-east England. Aside from labouring full-time as a parent to my siblings and I my mother worked as an Avon-lady, while my father, having worked down

---

[1] Shelley (1819). Original: "To the rich thou art a check, When his foot is on the neck". With respect to George Floyd (1973–2020) and Black Lives Matter.
[2] Huxley (1946).

J. P. Marshall (✉)
London, UK

© The Author(s), under exclusive license to Springer Nature Switzerland AG 2021
M. Milton (ed.), *Balancing on Quicksand*,
https://doi.org/10.1007/978-3-030-79136-0_2

the mines upon leaving school, then became a police officer. Adored, disciplined and comfortably acquiescent here to the demands of a divine sovereign promising immortality in paradise, when I was ten my parents, successful in their chosen careers and socially mobile, moved us to the new town of Washington. In some ways, this marked the end of my childhood. Thrown into a liminal space, distressing recurrent dreams involving the movement of time, space and matter first entered into my conscious experience. I would wake from these and my mother would find me sitting at the top of the stairwell outside my bedroom in a semi-conscious state of terror.

I understand these nightmares now as perhaps an early expression of ultimate concerns I endeavoured to keep from my conscious awareness, representative in existential terms of an early movement towards *authenticity*. Perhaps growing in awareness of the nothingness surrounding being, certainly progressively exploring my freedom by challenging rules, I commenced a career in shoplifting, understandable perhaps not only as a challenge to my father's Law but to the Law of my thrownness, my fallenness, my finitude. Perhaps also as a call to be seen by someone. Aged thirteen, on the cusp of surrendering my belief in a protective deity, I refused to continue to attend church with my family where we had communed all the weeks of our lives. Thenceforth my relationship with my father dissolved into a brawl of shaming insults, aggression and occasional violence mixed up for me with periods of homelessness, wandering the streets.

As these relationships fell apart, I ran into problems at my new school. I had settled in well enough to begin with, meeting gladly with measures of institutional "success" including high grades and personal success including making the football team and kissing girls. Matters developed when my affections for a girl the goalkeeper held a flame for were reciprocated with a kiss. And deteriorated when, egged on by his friends, the goalkeeper attacked me to find I fought back. Aged fourteen I had most of this team marching around school daily looking to fight me, and as I continued to fight back the continued assaults stirred up difficult feelings for me. I resorted to "playing truant", as they called it, though as "truancy" was defined as being out of school without good reason, it was not an unproblematic perspective on how I was responding to my situation. I was also chased bloodied and bruised by hoards outside of school, running into older boys who carried knives. And at some point, I too started carrying knives, including into school.

My sadness and fear masked by anger and contempt, I became in the eyes of others a "problem child"—"bad" to teachers and "mad" to peers. On the steadily diminishing occasions I chose to attend classes I became disruptive—revelling in a new and welcome kind of cognisance and acclaim that came with such disruption—and progressively came into conflict with authorities aggressively enforcing rules I met with ridicule. A narrative arose there was "something wrong" with me. I became convinced they were the ones who were mad. And when I was thrown out of school for good, I returned to wandering the streets, where I attached myself to a community of others; an enchanting coalescence of cocksure raconteurs from broken homes and better held oddballs also with something of the insurgency about them. Like myself, most of this insurgency seemed averse to the usual melodies and viewed by more convention-courting peers with desire, fear and curiosity, who increasingly courted them curiously for the LSD they sold, acid replacing alcohol as the drug of choice for many across this united kingdom that summer.

Abetted by my already fierce, though not yet fully ripe, opposition to authority, I made myself known in this kingdom, as psilocybin mushrooms and "dope" (hashish) were added to a kinship diet progressively increasing in states of many-splendoured bliss. Carnivals of hilarity, nonduality, comradeship and adventure that mostly unfurled while exploring, until dawn, streets, motorways and industrial estates. Before I graduated aged fifteen to ecstasy; conducive to dancing enraptured on the shooting star that was the UK's acid house and "rave" scene; sanctums so sublimely rich in communion that for a spell I felt myself heaven bound. I also stole to fund my connectivity with this communion, this heaven. We might see this, not only as an expression of opposition to the operation of oppressive power in my life, but also as a desire for meaning and belonging. Perhaps also as a response to the anxiety generated by repressed rage and sadness.

In spite of a promising launch to this parade of powders, pills and purple ohms these drugs, in time, began to accentuate my problems. Psychedelics particularly, at times, gave expression to emotional "devils": feelings and states I had learned to hide away. Over time in the wake of a handful of nightmarish journeys we might understand psychoanalytically as an expression of shadow material and existentially as increased confrontation with the givens of existence, my anxiety grew. Aged sixteen I was arrested for a street robbery I had taken part in leading to my first spell aged seventeen in prison, first her majesty's prison Durham—at a time when inmates spent at least twenty-three hours per day inside small, shared cells containing only beds and buckets for "slop out". Before I was transferred to a young offenders' institution where slashings, self-harm and the very bloody biting off of noses were the order of the day.

Shortly after turning eighteen, new to cocaine and struggling to cope with unremitting dread, I was referred by my GP to a psychiatrist. Though he did not share his diagnoses with me, this psychiatrist did put me on a succession of powerful "anti-psychotics" including risperidone and aripiprazole, commonly used to "treat" "schizophrenia" and "bipolar disorder", along with "mood stabilisers" including diazepam. Though in a sense I craved the ensuing zombification, I also now suspect this pathologising further entrenched the idea coping was synonymous with the ingestion of powerful drugs, foreclosing then any deeper, potentially more meaningful, examination of my "issues". Though I met with this psychiatrist intermittently for a time thereafter I do not recall he asked me in any depth about my story, this story. Our sessions were less an exchange, more a monologue on his part, primarily serving to magnify the feelings I had of being odd, alone and somehow fundamentally flawed.

Because the legislators of my youth and hence laws themselves had been rendered corrupt and ridiculous to me I became my own Law. And I checked, from the constitution of that Law, the "name of the father", "the big Other[3]", the prohibitive and punitive language of the fraternity into which I had been thrown. I refused further colonisation by an order I felt

---

[3] Lacan (1966).

had debased me on numerous levels, an order I came to think of disdainfully as "the system". The fellow hoodlums, thieves and lunatics making up my new order then became good objects, in opposition to any kind of authority figure—particularly members of the police and the church—as (hated) external bad objects. Being able to escape neither my distress nor the dictates of my culture entirely, I made drugs into good objects too, using from aged eighteen onwards not only prescribed psychiatric drugs but also street benzodiazepines and, increasingly, alcohol. This arsenal was used, too, to bring me down from my many "uppers". Choosing to get the hell out of Washington, I also sailed my chemical-laden ship up and down England and Scotland and in a headwind on to the Spanish Canary Islands where I sold ecstasy for two summers.

Though as I rounded these capes I had been ushered, over time, onto a chorus of cleaving edges, by oftentimes treacherous interior and exterior tides, it was only as I approached twenty-one that the severely leaky armada of offence I had become truly started to sink. Both in Spain and in the UK I would commonly "come to" in places I had never found myself before, sometimes hundreds of miles from where I last recalled finding myself. Often on a floor, sometimes in a bath or on a roof, a balcony, sometimes on or in a bed with a stranger or two, drugs and drugs paraphernalia and remnants of untold hours of chaos literally splattered across unrecognisable walls and ceilings. Sometimes in a field. A stairwell. Or a police cell. On occasion soaked in blood, piss or vomit, in a dizzying gale of uncertainty feeling a million miles from any previous version of myself or anything I could grasp as human. Mutilated and untethered, my entire being trembling violently, fingernails breaking on the fringe of an abyss.

I would endeavour mostly to remove that fringe before it swallowed me whole. A downer, less to "start the day" than to face the impending episode of "consciousness", as I could come to at any time in any given 24 hour period. Strong beer from a stranger's fridge and immodest doses of whisky would be optimal. I could be feeling stable—or at least taped up, held together—in minutes. I was often told I was charming. Charmingly I would empty the contents of whatever vessel of sedation I found, picking out cigarette butts from half-finished glasses, often retching and throwing up each time I took a swig and tried to keep the alcohol down.

And if no such avenues were open then brash or befuddled, I would transport myself to the nearest store, stealing what I could often when I had money in my pocket, which occasionally ended in a chase or a fight with a security guard and sometimes my arrest. Aged twenty-one, I entered a residential rehabilitation centre in the UK by the name of Phoenix House Tyneside on a court order. The order was I stay for a minimum of six months. I walked out after five and a half and was arrested following a police stop and search in the early hours of the following morning.

My hatred (of Law) and identity ("one opposed to Law") enabled me to cross judicial boundaries with ease, as a further rebuttal of the system I came to experience as an abuser inflicting multifarious forms of systemic and interpersonal violence upon its subjects. Inflictions evocative of earlier diminishing attitudes towards me, and which evoked similar responses: reproach and ridicule begot reproach and ridicule; aggression was met with aggression. I continued to hide myself. And my opposition to forms of constricting power compelled me deeper into recklessness. Awake for days one Sunday morning, for example, soon after trying to break down a heroin-broker's door armed with a kitchen knife, I found myself, bloodied, in the driving seat of a car I had stolen, high on cocaine, ecstasy, benzos and whisky, pursued at speed by a fleet of police vehicles as I hurled drugs I had been tasked to sell onto the motorway. Ultimately "fishtailed" by this fleet, I came to in the passenger seat, the car destroyed. Over time my increasingly troubled and troubling being not only attracted the steadfast attention of the authorities, but also irrevocably alienated most of my community of others, amounting to a further loss of my attachment figures. This process of these idealised compatriots distancing themselves felt particularly devastating. It might also be the case that unconsciously this was what I was choosing, through fear.

Over time, the stances of my culture towards me shaped my relationship with myself; over this period fashioning something like a superego into an internal saboteur. One of many reasons I continued for many years to use both prohibited and prescribed drugs was to stall an inner process of demolition; drugging as an attempt to silence interiorised persecutors; a tranquilisation of guilt and shame. My response to my situation over this time served to deny and conceal, in oblivion, in forgetting, this situation. My response also involved aggression and violence towards others; understandable not only as usually justified defence of my self, but also as defences against engagement with shame including projection of shame onto others, who were then attacked. Such violence was though also aimed at the self. In this sense it could be understood as a declaration of shame; an attack on a self felt deeply to be shameful. My response to my situation itself could be seen in this way: as self-attack, self-violence. A crusade to destroy the self, or at least disfigure it beyond absolution. This brings me back to my finitude.

Throughout this time, I sailed close to the edge, often. On basic levels, self-hatred, and my will to escape my situation, drove me to the edge of destroying myself. To die would mean avoiding ever having to fully feel emotions which felt unbearable; impossible. On another level such close dances afforded me a sense of having control over death; risk-taking as an active flirtation with death as part of my process of coming to terms with nothingness. My drug use also numbed the powerlessness I felt in relation to this nothingness. One late-Autumn night aged twenty-three I had perhaps my closest dance with nothingness. Pirouetting on the fringe, fleecing and fiddling most I met there, a lively troupe I had "de-drugged" freebooted me and, further roused by my effort to dance with them, proceeded to bludgeon me into stillness including by smashing a glass bottle into the back of my head. Leaving me lying unconscious and bleeding unstintingly into the ground, alone, in perhaps my most intimate embrace with that ground.

A "rock bottom" moment. Though really this period was a succession of rock bottom days, nights, weeks and months. Somewhere in the middle of it I scraped together an application to the rehab I had walked out of almost three years earlier. Near the nadir of it, a shadow, my togetherness directing me to the last haven of my mother's devotion, I was met with that devotion. Surrendering, I re-entered a liminal space tossing and convulsing, in which devils and madness violently and bloodily devoured me. I heard children singing the song "Show me the way to go home" ceaselessly. Not knowing then that these "voices" could be understood as split off youngsters within me crying out in hope, I became horrified, convinced by dominant ideas on these matters I had gone mad; perhaps the most scared I have ever been. One week later, through the worst of it and knowing I had for at least a short time been saved, I was arrested in my parents' home for a robbery I had taken part in months earlier on a motorway service station.

Bailed back to rehab, I met in that home, again, with a tower of selves hailing from the most deprived parts of these islands; from The Gorbals to Moss Side to the Shankill Road. I read. I wrote. I dreamt recurrently of beings chasing me. I felt remorse. Shame. I began to flourish. And when I travelled from rehab to Newcastle Crown Court six months later and the judge said "take him down" I smiled. Three and a half years is ok. I'm alive. Back in prison I ran a successful business, drawing portraits from photos of fellow inmates' families. I later studied counselling at college on day release. And following release aged twenty-six ticking the box marked "no" in response to the question of a criminal record I took a flight alone to Australia. I then travelled for four years including two years in India, largely on a motorbike. Still hiding myself, less with a death wish than before, I dipped my toes into the waters of Eastern philosophy and practices including yoga and vipassana meditation. I met with burning corpses and poverty. I fell in love with natures. I also hated. Despaired. Owned. Forgave. I became responsible, for my self, for Others. For my daughter, who called the foundations of my existence into question. Aged thirty-one I entered into university studies in South-East England where I spent most of fourteen years, also working as a care coordinator in drugs services in some of London's and Brighton's most disadvantaged areas. I shared seven years with a constellation of receptive consciousnesses; politically informed psychotherapists and counselling psychologists[4] who helped me to trust, and relate, as vessels for ushering me carefully into the unknown and forgotten. I became aware of my immortality projects.[5] I began making amends to, and salvaged my love for, my father, and my family, and elevated this love the more I learned of the battles they too have fought and fight due to the operation of

---

[4] Milton (2010) and Orlans with van Scoyoc (2008).
[5] Becker (1974).

power in their own lives. And the more I came to embrace my ethical responsibility in the face of the Other.[6] And perhaps also the big Other.

I partied over much of this post-prison period too, using a variety of drugs to help me through. I also became attuned over time to the processes shaping these acts—the roles played for example by culture, disavowal and my enduring opposition to Law. I grew mindful of the games I am playing including in relation to death. And slowly, over years, the more I tended responsibilities, and worked through and integrated states bound up with the past, the present and the givens of existence, the less I used these substances. I made a choice to hide from nothing. But not nothingness. And so for a time I put my masks down. As a wise man wrote, not everything faced can be changed, but nothing can be changed until faced.[7] I might add that in the company of holding Others, entheogens including MDMA, psilocybin, ayahuasca and hashish were conducive to this facing, removing boundaries and barriers, unlike alcohol and other prescribed drugs, which rather served often to forge and fortify them. Shaping my self into something akin to a panopticon. On this score, I also spent time on prescribed "antidepressants", which had their place, but ultimately interned both my emotions and my dreams, each pivotal in guiding me through my problems. Set free from that conundrum, I question the dogma people must render themselves powerless and abstemious to "successfully" "recover" from "addictions".

Telling my story has been key to my moving beyond. As has my meaning-making, thus inseparable from this story; I have over time applied different frameworks of understanding to my experiences. I have not, however, subscribed to dominant models of "addiction" as "illness" or "disease" that locate "it" reductively "in" the individual "addict" or "alcoholic", where difficulties in living are construed as stemming essentially from defects of self or character. I have come to believe rather that such struggles often stem from myriad life events and situations, including past and present abusive and neglectful relationships, trauma,

---

[6] Chanter (2010).
[7] Baldwin (1962). Original: "Not everything that is faced can be changed; but nothing can be changed until it is faced".

racism, sexism, bereavement, bullying, gender expectations, economic pressures and more existential challenges such as finding meaning in uncertainty and isolation. In times of corruption, injustice and ubiquitous abuse of political and ideological power, the manifold bitter fruits of which include racial and class oppression, xenophobia, devastating austerity and inequality, poverty, status anxiety and the continued destruction of nature in the face of the unfolding climate and ecological emergency, it seems to me that conceptualisations of the self as innately "sick" often serve to overshadow and annul potentially more helpful meaning-making.[8] Misleading many of us so categorised into believing these labels reflect the existence at the root of our suffering of chronic, biological diseases and "chemical imbalances", best "treated" with "medication[9]" and CBT.[10] The dominant tradition dictating how we approach phenomena so as to close off certain questions. Such dictates to make people fixed could be seen as dictates to deny dizzying freedom. Midwives of bad faith. Endeavours to unsee a painful or inconvenient reality one sees. A deformation or evasion of one's or another's choice of who one or another will be.

While I believe there are limits to choice and to transcendence of facticity, I do not believe I am powerless in relation to "addiction." I have not allowed my baggage to define my being. I am consoled by the assertion a human being is not yet a self, implying as it does that ontologically we are in a constant state of becoming. I do not see my past behaviour as indicative of fixed pathologies, but increasingly as meaning-based survival strategies, threat responses.[11] I have come to believe that the industry of arbitrarily deciding what pathology is and is not, without a basis in science or evidence, is an intrinsically political endeavour, serving to preserve the interests of those in power. A violence to the irreducible plurality, singularity and uncertainty of the Other.

---

[8] Marshall (2021).
[9] Moncrieff (2020).
[10] Loewenthal and Proctor (2019) and Rizq (2011).
[11] Boyle and Johnstone (2020) and Johnstone et al. (2018).

I have learned that beneath the layers of my conditioning there lies not badness, madness or illness as Others would have me believe, but beautiful things, which now shine when seen.

For a long time, I feared if I looked deeply within, I would find something corrupt, sick, evil, a monster. For a long time, I held back pain bound up with my past, through fear of disintegration, which amounted to a holding back of my self. For a long time, I held back my younger selves, when my younger selves are my power. Later in time, older, kinder, politically active, a psychotherapist training as a counselling psychologist, a loving father, telling myself as I danced and sang one day that I had come so far; it struck me I had a lot to thank my younger selves for. I felt in that dance and song the pain of the worst of those times. I felt myself, breathing deeply, shuddering, returned to the past in myriad forms. Opening. And I stopped dancing, sat down and sobbed. And I viewed these weeping selves through the prism of the person I am now. I held them. Holding myself. Accepted them. Accepting myself. Forgave them. Forgiving myself. Loved them. Loving myself. I saw no evil in or among them. No monsters. I saw an artist. A player. A fighter. A dreamer. A friend. Love. I saw pathways through time. And I sobbed much of my pain out. I had kept these selves at a distance as I had feared their pain might hurt me. They had kept me apart as they had feared I would let them down, abandon them, as Others had; those Others often abandoned too. But no, I accepted them. And they trusted me. In reality, this coalescence has given me the most responsibility. What I feared might cause my disintegration has led to my elevation. Children's songs no longer split off, or sedated, but part of me. Unified. Empowered. Still pushing. Home.

References

Baldwin, J. (1962). As much truth as one can bear. *New York Times Book Review, 14*, 2.

Becker, E. (1974). *The denial of death*. Simon and Schuster.

Boyle, M., & Johnstone, L. (2020). *A straight talking introduction to the power threat meaning framework. An alternative to psychiatric diagnosis.* PCCS Books.

Chanter, T. (Ed.). (2010). *Feminist interpretations of Emmanuel Levinas.* Penn State University Press.

Huxley, A. (1946). *Foreword to second edition of Brave new world (1932).* HarperCollins.

Johnstone, L., & Boyle, M., with Cromby, J., Dillon, J., Harper, D., Kinderman, P., Longden, E., Pilgrim, D., & Read, J. (2018). *The Power Threat Meaning Framework: Towards the identification of patterns in emotional distress, unusual experiences and troubled or troubling behaviour, as an alternative to functional psychiatric diagnosis.* British Psychological Society.

Lacan, J. (1966). *Écrits* (B. Fink, Trans.). Norton.

Loewenthal, D., & Proctor, G. (2019). *Why not CBT? Against and for CBT revisited.* PCCS Books.

Marshall, J. P. (2021). *Toward a psychology of (un)certainty. An interpretative phenomenological analysis of young people's accounts of receiving a diagnosis of bipolar disorder* (Doctoral thesis, Regent's University London).

Milton, M. (Ed.) (2010). *Therapy and beyond: Counselling psychology contributions to therapeutic and social issues.* Wiley-Blackwell.

Moncrieff, J. (2020). *A straight talking introduction to psychiatric drugs: The truth about how they work and how to come off them* (2nd ed.). PCCS Books.

Orlans, V. with van Scoyoc, S. (2008). *A short introduction to counselling psychology.* Sage.

Rizq, R. (2011). The perversion of care: Psychological therapies in a time of IAPT. *Psychodynamic Practice, 18* (1), 7–24.

Shelley, P. B. (1819). *The masque of anarchy.* Retrieved from http://knarf.eng lish.upenn.edu/PShelley/anarchy.html.

Breaking the Rules

Alison Greenwood

I've just finished a telephone call with the mother of a 24-year-old client who began the conversation with "*I know I shouldn't have phoned, but…*". It's 7:45 pm on a Friday evening, I'm concerned for my client, I'm ready for a glass of wine, and I'm wondering how many professional boundaries I've just crashed through. Again. She's right of course, she shouldn't have phoned, and I shouldn't have answered, I'm not a crisis number, it wasn't a crisis, she's not even my client, and it could certainly have waited until Monday. However, I judge it to have been a helpful call, I was able to reduce both her anxiety and her daughter's, so why am I left feeling defensive about my behaviour?

I am a counselling psychologist, so I have been trained to think relationally and to be reflective: I assess, once again, whether this could be as much about meeting my own needs as it was about meeting my client's; I ask myself, once again, what's in it for me when I "go the extra mile"?

A. Greenwood (✉)
Richmond, UK
e-mail: alison@doseofnature.org.uk

I wonder, once again, whether I am resilient enough to sit with my own feelings of inadequacy, if I feel I have not done everything I possibly can for a client; and most importantly, I consider, *once again*, whether there has been, or could potentially be in future, any adverse effect on my client of this boundary transgression. I reflect, and I conclude that there was therapeutic benefit in my out of hours contact with the mother of my client; I may have been unboundaried in answering the call, but in this particular case, with this particular set of circumstances, I did what was in the best interests of my client; it was helpful and caused no harm, either to myself or my client. And that's my conclusion. Reflection done, client helped, glass of wine deserved. But, of course, it is not that easy and questions arise before I have taken my first sip. Will the mother take advantage of my immediate availability? How can I be sure my client agreed to her mother's intervention? And since I cannot guarantee this level of access, what are the consequences if I don't pick up next time?

Boundaries are not a straight-forward concept for anyone new to therapy, whichever side of the therapeutic encounter you sit. A therapist/client relationship is unlike any other. It is frequently acknowledged as the most important factor in the effectiveness of therapy, and yet its complex and often unfamiliar nature, at least on the part of the client, gives rise to the potential for harm on both sides. A set of "tried and tested" rules then, guiding and governing the behaviour of both therapist and client, seems an eminently sensible way to ensure the protection of both. Indeed, professional bodies such as the British Psychological Society (BPS) have produced practice guidelines and codes of conduct that include information which is extremely helpful, and across a wide range of therapeutic modalities, and with surprisingly few exceptions, there is broad consensus as to what constitutes "good practice" in terms of maintaining professional boundaries. However, the professional bodies do not stipulate blind adherence to a rigid set of rules, but rather are at pains to point out that "*no guidance can replace the need for psychologists to use their own judgement*[1]". And therein lies my troubled relationship with the recognised rules of therapy. The concept of boundaries is undeniably a good one, based on a sound rationale to protect both client

---

[1] BPS (2018).

and therapist, but boundaries are not legal requirements, or at least the ones under discussion here are not,[2] and as such are open to challenge and interpretation. What follows then is a personal account of situations that have arisen in my own practice where I have found myself blurring, stretching, or completely disregarding recognised therapeutic boundaries, and an honest discussion of the consequences, both positive and negative, of these transgressions. With little attempt to provide clear answers, I ask the same questions I have been asking over ten years of practice: does adhering to therapeutic boundaries always lead to the most effective therapeutic outcomes? Is 'best practice" sometimes in conflict with what is best for clients? And are there times when we should consider *"breaking the rules"*?

I first encountered the term "therapeutic boundary" at a bereavement counselling training course, when we were told that accepting an offered cup of tea on a visit to a bereaved client would constitute "a boundary violation". I remember politely enquiring after the rationale for behaviour that appeared so unfriendly and so unnatural, and I recollect our trainer explaining the therapeutic frame, and the importance of an agreed set of rules that served to protect both client and counsellor, that maintained clarity, and would avoid any future confusion or misunderstandings about the nature of the relationship: clear expectations in the form of explicit boundaries helped the client and therapist to feel in control and were experienced as reassuring by both parties. That all made sense and sounded entirely sensible — but a cup of tea? Really? Did that affect the frame to such an extent that it could cause harm to the client or adversely affect the relationship? I really wanted to understand, but I kept coming back to the first session of the course where we had learnt that building a trusting, caring relationship was central to effective counselling. That had also made complete sense, but now I was faced with a "boundary" that I felt could potentially jeopardise that relationship in the first few minutes of meeting. I remember suggesting to our tutor, who on reflection was incredibly patient with me, that *surely* turning down an offered cup of tea would, at best, miss out on an early opportunity to

---

[2] Boundary issues relating to a therapist's legal obligations with regards to data protection, safeguarding, health & safety, and sexual exploitation are not a feature of this discussion.

create a warm and friendly environment in which to build trust, and at worst, risk offending the client before we had even sat down.

Ten years later, and I now understand the wider implications of accepting an offered drink: the power dynamics it can set up from the outset, the unwelcome distraction it can cause at the beginning of a session and the potential confusion it can create about the nature of the relationship. In my current role, I still sometimes see clients in their own homes, but I almost always refuse a cup of tea, for what I now recognise to be sound therapeutic reasons, and yet just occasionally I accept, in spite of my understanding, because just occasionally, all things considered and duly reflected upon, I judge it to be the right thing to do. And sometimes I'm just thirsty.

As a trainee psychologist, my boundary violations were a recurrent theme in my supervision sessions. I was keen to understand why it was so ill-advised to accept a gift or receive a hug or lend a book? Boundaries around time were my most frequent transgressions. I struggled to understand why if a client arrived 15 minutes late "with good reason", I could not see them for the full hour if I was available to do so, or why it mattered so much if I allowed a session to run over a little with a client who had "one more thing to say". How could these small acts of kindness towards a person in distress be "wrong"? And, like the cup of tea, I wondered about the potential negative impact of disappointing a vulnerable client who had their gift rejected, or hug refused, or was coldly told they could not attend their therapy session at all if they had arrived 20 minutes late. As a trainee, I listened to the individual rationales for these boundaries and was largely convinced by the potential harm that seemingly small transgressions of this kind can cause, setting up false expectations that cannot be maintained, or undermining the professional quality of the relationship. I also came to understand the therapeutic merit of disappointing a client or holding them to account for their behaviour. Then one day a client, who had always been early for sessions, arrived in a fluster 25 minutes late, explaining that she had been unable to find anywhere to park. She was extremely apologetic and very stressed, and, against instinct, I upheld the service's rule that we should not see someone who arrived more than 15 minutes late. The client was devastated, she burst into tears, left the therapy room and did not return.

My supervisor was kind but challenged a decision I had described as "against instinct". Why had I not followed my own judgement? I was training to be a professional psychologist and I needed the confidence to question boundaries when they were not in the best interests of my client. My adherence to the service's rule had been the wrong decision for this client at this moment and caused her to disengage from therapy. I learnt a valuable lesson: the boundaries established by organisations may not always be in the best interests of our clients.

For two of my three trainee years, I was fortunate enough to have two excellent supervisors with whom I felt comfortable and safe enough to explore the various boundaries I had tip-toed over, or marched straight through. In discussions with them, I gained insight into my behaviour, particularly in respect of my "wanting to do more", and I came to a clearer understanding of the consequences, positive and negative, for both me and my clients, of the situations where I had pushed or crossed a boundary. Most importantly though, with these wise and experienced supervisors, I began to see each situation as unique, and each one worthy of individual exploration. I came to distinguish between rules and guidelines, and between those that were in the best interests of the client, those that protected the therapist, and those that served the organisation. We discussed how useful boundaries could be if properly understood and thoughtfully applied, but also the potential for them to be harmful if given precedence over a therapist's judgement. I learnt that every therapeutic encounter has an individual set of circumstances, and while acknowledging "good practice" and established protocols, effective decisions should never be made without reference to these particular circumstances. My supervisors gave me the confidence to trust my own judgement and set me free to be the therapist I wanted to be. I learnt by making mistakes: I often got things wrong, but I learnt because I felt safe enough to share these mistakes with my supervisors.

My third supervisor taught me another important lesson. She had a psychoanalytic background and modelled strict boundaries in our supervision sessions together, but I was afraid of her judgement and would rarely share my boundary dilemmas, let alone confess to any transgressions. As a practitioner with a tendency towards stretching boundaries and a desire to experiment with different ways of working, I soon came to understand the importance of an open and trusting supervisory relationship once I no longer had it. Breaking the rules, I came to realise, was a lot harder, and unquestionably riskier, without someone I trusted to talk to.

Shortly, after qualifying as a psychologist, I crossed a new boundary: I saw a client outside of therapy. The client in question was a young man who was extremely insecure and suffered from chronic anxiety. At school, he had been a keen actor and had played leading roles in school plays. When he was 18 and in his first year at university he suffered a traumatic experience that led to a suicide attempt, he dropped out of university and was referred to our services for therapy. When we first met, he was spending 15–20 hours a day in bed and was rarely leaving the house. Over the course of therapy, his confidence increased, and he joined an amateur dramatics club. It was towards the end of his allotted six months of therapy that he invited me to go and watch his play. I was hesitant and feared that my current supervisor would not approve, but I felt it might be helpful. My client and I agreed we would not acknowledge each other when he was with his family, and I would see the play and leave immediately afterwards. I reflected on my reasons for wanting to go … Was I afraid of disappointing him? Did I want him to like me more, or be grateful for my commitment? I reflected and I concluded: my motives were therapeutic, and in my client's best interests. I hoped my going would be validation that he was worth something, and that he had formed a meaningful relationship with someone who genuinely cared. I anticipated being able to praise his performance in our next therapy session and looked forward to the further confidence boost that might give him. I also reflected on any potential harm: false expectations of a future relationship, a lack of professionalism undermining our future work, a dependency that might make our imminent ending more difficult, and I concluded that in this particular case with this particular person, it was the right thing to do. My supervisor was sceptical, but held a view based on her own experience of therapy, admittedly far greater than mine, but based on "most people" in "most contexts", and I felt my experience in this particular case was greater than hers, so I trusted my own judgement, and saw the play. My client was very good, and in our next session together he was beaming. I had witnessed his triumph and that had been of huge benefit to his confidence, but it was the fact that I had gone at all that had been of greatest therapeutic benefit—in being prepared to see him outside of the therapy room, in a role other than as a client, I was showing him that I trusted him, respected him and valued him for the person he was. It is certainly not a practical way to behave with every client, it would not be appropriate, and might cause harm, but in this case, our therapy ended successfully three weeks later, and in the thank you card he handed me as we parted, he had written simply, "that meant a lot".

Some of my boundary transgressions are more straightforward than others. I certainly don't always get it right, but when I don't, I usually recognise, on reflection or in supervision, that I haven't. However, occasionally, this is not the case and I am left unclear as to whether my unboundaried behaviour was helpful or harmful. When this happens, I am reminded that people are complex, and their behaviour full of contradictions and inconsistencies, so it is hardly surprising that an attempt to impose rigid rules on relationships gives rise to so many dilemmas, uncertainties and questions.

A particularly controversial situation for me arose when I accompanied a client to court. The client was appealing a previous court decision in which she had lost custody of her child following an earlier psychotic episode. Since this isolated episode, she had made a full recovery, completed six months of therapy with me, been medication-free for over a year, and was, in both my judgement and that of the consultant psychiatrist, not only safe to take care of her young son, but capable of providing him with a loving and nurturing environment in which to thrive. Beyond a letter to the judge, our psychiatrist was keen for us "not to get involved", but I felt compelled to do all I could to support her. I wasn't asked to testify, but I requested to do so, and this had given my client hope that she would win. On the morning of the trial, I picked her up and sat next to her in court. We were both feeling confident. I was a professional and she trusted me, and she had spent three months believing that she would be reunited with her son. But she wasn't, the judge considered my evidence to be biased, and the independent psychiatrist, on the basis of a 45-minute assessment concluded that the diagnosis was one from which a full recovery was unlikely.

The written evidence from the client's own psychiatrist describing the recovery was also deemed insufficiently objective to overrule the court's expert. My client was left devasted and feeling utterly let down; she left our service that day and never returned, her trust in our service irrevocably broken. I was deemed to have been too involved, and to have not maintained appropriate professional boundaries. Some years later, I now wonder whether, had I not attended court that day as my supervisor and the psychiatrist had advised, the judgement may have been the same, but this vulnerable young mother would not have had the same expectations of a positive outcome, and may not have lost faith with services that might have been helpful to her in future. But at the same time as wondering whether, on this occasion, I did indeed "*go too far*", I find myself also questioning whether in fact I went far enough. I had felt inhibited by professional boundaries and not acted instinctively. Should I have talked to her solicitor? Should I have encouraged our service to have greater involvement? Should I have submitted a report on delusional disorder? Should I in fact have done *more*?

In life, "going the extra mile" is usually a good thing, but in the world of therapy, I have frequently encountered criticism for behaviour that I have judged simply to be kind, helpful and supportive. Of course, I understand the risks and potential harm to clients that some unboundaried behaviour can cause, but if we are going to get the balance wrong sometimes, and of course we all will, I wonder if it is better to get it wrong by being too kind, and caring too much, rather than being too detached, and caring too little. As a newly qualified psychologist, who had often been told to care a little less, I remember being delighted to read research that notes that clients particularly value a sense that they really matter to their therapist, and "*service beyond expectation*" was found to be a significant factor in therapeutic success.[3]

I once visited a client at home who said he was too low to come to the hospital where we usually met. He was a recovering alcoholic, and his wife was extremely worried about him relapsing. I had been seeing him for two months, although his attendance had been patchy, and he seemed at risk of disengaging. However, my visit marked a turning point

---

[3] Cooper (2018).

in our relationship, and he went on to successfully complete six months of therapy without missing another session. On another occasion, I got involved in a disabled client's housing appeal, leaving messages on her housing officer's answering machine every day for three weeks. After five years of not being able to leave her home unless she had a friend there to help her down the stairs, she was finally rehoused to a ground floor flat and was able to take daily walks independently. It is hard to argue with the accusation that I was acting beyond my role, and I acknowledge it had little to do with therapy, but those persistent two-minute messages at the beginning of my day had a far greater impact on this client's life than all our therapy sessions put together. During my time as a therapist, I have posted books, made birthday cakes, sent cards and lent DVDs, all of which might reasonably be considered unboundaried behaviour, and certainly "against the rules" in many services, but the extent to which these actions were "wrong" is, perhaps, a more difficult question.

Over the course of my ten years of practice, sometimes I have been faced with rules that have appeared to protect neither client nor therapist, but rather served the best interests of the organisation. Of course, an organisation's regulations are a vital part of keeping everyone safe, but sometimes I wonder if a little more flexibility and a more trusting attitude towards conscientious professionals would enable more effective practice. In particular, I have experienced numerous occasions when risk-management principles have taken precedence over humane interventions, with negative consequences for the client that might easily have been avoided if a less rigid approach had been adopted. On one occasion, a client whom I had been seeing for over three months and with whom I had a good relationship, started a new job and asked if it would be possible for us to have an early appointment before his work. He was in the middle of therapy and did not want to stop something that was having a positive impact on his life, but he also did not want to ask for time off work or disclose to his new colleagues that he was having therapy. I always arrived at work at 8am and shared with my manager my willingness to arrive fifteen minutes earlier to start a session at 7:45 in order to accommodate my client's request. However, no amount of petitioning moved my manager from her steadfast position that it was simply not permissible on grounds of personal safety. I knew my client well and was angry that my personal judgement was being overridden in such a senseless way. The client dropped out of therapy and I was in no doubt that the potential for helping this person had been missed on account of too rigid an adherence to rules. But then again, …

It was less than six months later when a colleague ignored their service's lone working policy and called at the home of one her clients, whom she also claimed to know well, in response to a mother's concern for her son's erratic behaviour. On her arrival, she was led through to the garden by the mother and left to speak with her client, who immediately pulled a knife from his jacket and stabbed his therapist. Fortunately, she was not badly injured, but the incident was a timely reminder to me that some rules should not be broken lightly.

I've worked as a therapist in a variety of different contexts, in the NHS, the third sector, schools, private practice, and now I run a charity that promotes the mental health benefits of engaging with nature, and I work with clients, unsurprisingly, outdoors. Boundary requirements have changed significantly according to a whole range of factors—different physical environments, different organisational structures, different client groups and different manager and supervisor styles, and now, within the limits of a professional ethical framework, I am free to set my own rules. However, the sense of liberation I expected to feel, no longer constrained by the strict boundaries imposed by others, has not materialised: it seems that writing my own rules is much more difficult than breaking other people's. Working in an outdoor setting with no four walls to provide physical containment, and with a host of unpredictable factors to consider, such as the weather, other people, animals, noise, I am in no doubt that whatever parameters I might want to put in place for myself and others to follow, principles of flexibility and adaptability need to be prioritised. Unexpected things are more likely to happen when outside the therapy room and instinctive quick decisions that do not necessarily follow recognised therapeutic boundaries are frequently required. I have had a client cling on to me in terror as we negotiated a particularly aggressive dog; I have taken a client to hospital in my car with a suspected broken ankle; and my therapeutic hour has doubled after getting lost in a forest. Working outside I have developed a more practical approach to therapy, and faced with new situations on a regular basis, I am constantly updating and rethinking our rules. Recently, I learnt that there is a freedom and informality about being outside that can confuse a relationship: I met a client new to our service at a local park on a beautiful sunny day and after just a few minutes walking by a lake, the client turned to me and said "this seems like a date, I don't want to spoil it by telling you my problems"! Hmm? I'm not sure I have an answer as to how to reduce the risk of this kind of confusion in future. Should I try to make a walk outside in a beautiful natural setting less lovely? Should I create some *new* rules? Increase formality? Be less warm? Stick to cloudy days and boring landscapes? None of these are appealing propositions, and in reality, I'm unlikely to change my approach, but the incident highlights the unexpected challenges this new way of working presents, and the need to adopt a pragmatic and flexible approach to issues of boundary as they arise.

Wouldn't it be wonderful if following the rules were as straightforward as the instructions given to Alice, "*Read the directions, and directly you will be directed in the right direction*[4]", and breaking the rules were as exhilarating as Hermione Granger suggests, "*It's sort of exciting, isn't it, breaking the rules*[5]"? However, my own experiences have taught me that whether following the rules or breaking them, it is never simple and rarely fun, but rather it is complex and confusing, and often difficult and distressing. And if I have any conclusion at all to offer, it is that "acting with compassion", "being mindful of context" and "using common sense", are the guiding principles I have learned to value most when judging whether a boundary might be usefully respected, or transgressed.

References

British Psychological Society. (2018). *Code of ethics and conduct*. British Psychological Society. https://www.bps.org.uk/sites/www.bps.org.uk/files/Policy/Policy%20-%20Files/BPS%20Code%20of%20Ethics%20and%20Conduct%20%28Updated%20July%202018%29.pdf.

---

[4] Carrol (1920).
[5] Yates (2007).

Carroll, L. (1920). *Alice's adventures in wonderland*. Macmillan.
Cooper, M. (2008). *Essential research findings in counselling and psychotherapy*. Sage.
Yates, D. (Director). (2007). *Harry Potter and the order of the Phoenix* [Film]. Warner Brothers Pictures.

Disturbing the Peace: Madame X vs Westminster Council

Martin Milton

Message to the audience: *"Westminster Council has a very strict policy of not disturbing the peace, of stopping shows before 11 pm. Should artists not comply, the plug will be pulled, the safety curtain will be dropped"*. Literally. Dissension is not possible. Peace must be maintained at all costs.

Not a bad rule. But a rule all the same and not completely commensurate with the artistic and creative energies of performers and the two thousand plus people who gather in the theatre.

Artists are here to disturb the peace.

It's February 2020, a cold Wednesday night in London. One icon quotes another. The Queen of Pop referencing James Baldwin. The exquisitely conceived and choreographed show is running late—not hours late, but maybe 5 or 10 minutes. Will she make it or do we all have to be good

---

M. Milton (✉)
Regent's University London, London, UK
e-mail: miltonm@regents.ac.uk

© The Author(s), under exclusive license to Springer Nature
Switzerland AG 2021
M. Milton (ed.), *Balancing on Quicksand*,
https://doi.org/10.1007/978-3-030-79136-0_4

and shut down early? Be quiet and go home? Do as we are told and follow the rules?

There is a particular irony to events tonight. This isn't your run of the mill "pop concert", but rather, we are told, a full-blown expression of artistic concern. It spotlights inequality, gun ownership, misogyny and sexual violence, and how these are all facilitated by the status quo, by not speaking up, by letting power run wild. Change needs to come we are told, but it can only come through a disruption of the peace. The gun laws cannot be taken as acceptable. Misogyny mustn't be seen as normal, nor racism, colonialism or any lauding of power over others.

To demand the artist cut 5 minutes off a show simply to meet the "peacefulness" rule is unrealistic. No wonder the Queen of Pop calls Bullshit on that. Actually she calls "Censorship"—it amounts to the same thing.

Time slips. We are almost at the end of the playlist, but that doesn't matter. The sound system is turned off. The atmosphere is charged ...

Does that work? No, of course it doesn't. The audience experiences it as a silencing, an impediment to thinking critically. It fuels tonight's call to *Rise Up* and to engage.

The stage lights are turned off, and the auditorium lights turned on. It's an experience of dictatorship (albeit constructed as benevolent in intent, at least for the highly privileged neighbours). The unnamed "they" assume *they* must, should and will tell you what you can see and when. Did they really think this would work? It was never going to, not here, not tonight. This is an audience drawn explicitly to a critique of power. People aren't going anywhere just because some rule-abiding agent of the council flicks a switch or two.

So, what that we can no longer hear the Queen of Pop without her mic? No problem! We'll all sing *for* her! She can no longer perform atop her expensively built stage. So what? A passionate sing-along in front of the dropped curtain means more to the audience than the Council could ever imagine. And keeps us there. We rise up! We face down this provocation. It turns the audience from observers of art to disturbers of the peace, activists in their quest for imaginative and social justice.

Artists are here to disturb the peace. Otherwise, chaos.[1]

These issues are much broader than the case of Madame X vs Westminster Council. They go to the heart of who can speak and who not? Who sets the rules and who abides by them? Power games like this play out in domestic and social spheres, they're seen in the office, poisoning relationships between communities and Nation States too.[2] They prowl social media and are evident in the ways that we gaslight the lives of so many.

For far too long, racial, sexual and gendered minorities have been overlooked, silenced and subject to personal and systemic abuse through "reasonableness". Rule following needs to be combined with an ability to change them when they are unfair or unjust. Many of the rules we abide by need resetting. Coronavirus, the killing of George Floyd and the #MeToo movement have shown us this too.

Like James Baldwin and Madonna, John Lewis the US Congressman called for change, suggested a disruption of injustice, from atop the Edmund Petrus Bridge in Selma, Alabama. He enjoined us to "Get in good trouble, necessary trouble, and help redeem the soul of America[3]". Lewis' was such an exquisitely crafted call—No one can argue that there is an urgent, moral and ethical case to dismantle the systemic racism that poisons societies around the world. But his call also asks us to think about what constitutes good disruption and what constitutes bad?

It's not only our heroes that disrupt, across the world we are seeing disruption becoming the leadership style of the day. We see abrupt, forceful disruption, delight being taken in partisanship and we see money and power coming together to disrupt expectations of the rule of law[4] and democracy. Political appointments lead to outrage but, in the short term at least, remain. The US Environmental Protection Agency was led by men who were proudly anti-environmental regulation. In the UK, there is concern as the Prime Minister appoints acolyte disrupters to

---

[1] Literary Conversations Series (Undated).
[2] These issues are front and centre in The Police, Crime, Sentencing and Courts Bill 2021 before Parliament as I write this.
[3] Thorne (2020).
[4] See investigations of Roger Stone in the US, or the UK Supreme Court ruling on the illegality of proroguing Parliament.

key cabinet posts; why have a committed climate expert at the helm of COP26? Just add it as a *second* portfolio for someone that has frequently voted against environmental protections. Why appoint an experienced Attorney General, one who works well with the judiciary when you can have a relative newcomer writing that Parliament has "ceded power" to the courts, and this should be "retrieved[5]". And Parliament is asked to vote for legislation that, even the government proposers, agree breaks international law. Disruption can be a key political tool.[6]

The case of Madame X vs Westminster Council sheds light on another interesting aspect, and that's the issue of *how* we scrutinise and police the status quo. Of course, there is a whole web of mechanisms supporting the powerful, but one is particularly surprising. Often, the policing of the peace is delegated to those low on the power ladder, often those on minimum wages. And this is not accidental as when we have little power, we are concerned not to lose what we have, or at least not to incur the wrath of the powerful. The theatre's reaction to Madame X's running over was to enforce the rule quickly, underlings becoming ardent enforcers of the rules. They need their jobs. But did they maybe also enjoy the power? Psychoanalysis has long helped us understand the powerful phenomenon termed "identification with the aggressor[7]". It's that process whereby we get a tiny, delicious, taste of power by adjoining myself with the powerful, it is itself a disruption. It disrupts the stark awareness of the pain of powerlessness we experience in other circumstances.

Maybe it is also a chance to get back at the powerful woman on stage and try to make her follow the rules? A woman who is known to have little truck with gendered and sexual prohibition. Who does she think she is?

---

[5] Conservatives at Home (2020).

[6] And of course, this isn't new - governments have long set brutal, intrusive scrutinising rules. The preoccupation with stopping benefit recipients ("scroungers") claiming a penny more than they are entitled to ("deserve"), all the while playing fast and loose with parliamentary expenses and letting corporations away with paying miniscule amounts of the tax are just some obvious examples at the political level.

[7] Howell (2014).

While underlings turn off sound systems, or in the case of the benefits system scrutinise claims with far greater vigour than checking their own bank statements, we hear of rule-setters taking "donations" from all and sundry, claiming unrealistic expenses, limiting their work so as to hold down multiple jobs, and play by a completely different set of rules. The country goes in to lockdown yet the powerful break the rules with very little sanction.

How come? The status quo is powerful. Power begets power we are told. The coming together of powerful allies and serious resources is important too, and of course, those that desire an ethical, transparent code of social practice are hampered by not being able to utilise some of the nastier, more insidious forms of disruption available to others.

Can it change? Should it change? These are long-standing questions that play out internationally, nationally and in our interpersonal relations. But one thing is for sure, change never happens through more of the same.

With censorship, silencing and invisibilising comes a diminishment, a lack of possibility and great damage both socially and psychically. Without the freedom to express ourselves, to exist, comes distress, no matter whether that emanates through restrictive government policy, or the denial of self, intended to avoid stigma. And this is where psychotherapists enter the fray.

And fray it is. The ethics and science of our own profession require us to understand the individual, help shed some light on personal and social dilemmas and consider ways to accept or change circumstance so as to escape oppression.

While we do this in the consulting room with small numbers—individuals, couples and groups, it is also true that psychotherapeutic experience, expertise and knowledge offer broader insights. We hear about the impact of the gender pay gap, see the damage of systemic racism, work with life-threatening homophobia and transphobia. And we see the damage it does to us all—victims obviously, but perpetrators too.

While we may be comfortable in our consulting rooms it is important for members of the psy-professions to join the conversations and add our voices alongside those we serve. We shouldn't claim a singular entitlement, nor overstate the impact of our knowledge, but neither should we shy away from offering insight as to the damage that the status quo is doing. Power structures are complicit in causing and maintaining the inequalities that lead to depression, to anxiety, stress and suicidality.

Another reason for us to reflect critically is that, as with everything else, our profession is subject to scrutiny and control, sometimes helpfully, often very unhelpfully. Rigid understandings of "evidence bases" forced upon us, manualisation, the imposition of time limits as if all our clients are "standard" clients guaranteed to respond in the same way at the same pace.

We shouldn't resist such views simply for the sake of resistance, because there may well be a place for these policies for *some* people *some* of the time. The dilemma is more complex. Very little of what is fetishised as an evidence base informs the practicing psychotherapist as to what will help *this* client, with their *particular* circumstances. On the contrary, there is real, incontrovertible evidence for the tailoring of the therapeutic relationship to specific clients and their unique needs.

The oppression that leads to a person's distress is seldom worked into a manualised therapy, it's often not evident in policies developed in the age of austerity either. The assumption of personal frailty, or faulty ways of thinking doesn't capture the fact that distress is as much a function of a racist, homophobic or misogynistic culture, rooted in our socio-economic preoccupations as it may be the result of internalised familial trauma. Oppression can be subtle and absorbed over a long time as well as sometimes dramatic and identifiable as one traumatic event. Depression is often a sense of powerlessness—being trapped, opportunity vanished, options limited.[8] To express one's frustration, despair or upset directly feels impossible. Anxiety[9] too is often exacerbated by a worry about the disaster that awaits should one not *do* the right thing or *be* the right thing. And we have seen, over recent years, models of mental health care can exacerbate this. Insurance companies tell *you*

---

[8] See Gilbert (2017).

[9] For a thought provoking and sensitive look at anxiety, see May (1977).

whether you warrant therapy or not. They claim their methods are in your interest—but are they?

It certainly doesn't always feel like they are. The gracious "offer" of 6 sessions is an insult to the deep distress experienced and constitutes a pressure to conform. Organisations offer several sessions of "counselling" if you are upset about a restructuring and being made redundant. The requirement of a diagnosis to access a service turns one's need to express oneself into a pathology, you are no longer expressing powerlessness in the face of damaging circumstances but evidencing your depressive character traits or your negative thoughts. They back this up with an evidence base that is frequently over-stated and poorly attuned. In these models, no longer is the therapist expected to be attuned, to think, to accompany the client on a tailored way through their tribulations in life. No they are there simply to follow the rules because, apparently, the writers of the rules know what will do YOU, specifically, the best. What is often missing is the relational, the reflection on the impact of policies on the public.

This means that members of the psy-complex find themselves having to manage the dilemma of disruption too. Diagnose, follow the manual, and encourage people back into work by following the rules? OR help your client find their voice? This isn't new. The history of psychotherapy is one of disruption—just read Jung, Laing, Freud or Rogers with an eye to the times. The psychotherapist is—or should be—an artist, their medium, the psyche.

If psychotherapists are to act with others as more than agents of the state, as scrutinisers of the status quo, we may have to be disruptive, to find our voices and use them. And this is ethical. As Susie Orbach so ably noted, no matter what the machine says "we have the authority of what we hear clinically. We know how to think about the psychological and social damage that is done to individuals and families by the society we all inhabit and actively engage with[10]". We have access to the truth of an individual's experience in a way that governments, statisticians and algorithms do not. They cannot.

---

[10] Starkman (2015).

Before the anxious rule followers get too worried—I am not suggesting that this is license for therapists to run riot, do what we like as some of the more grotesque political examples of the past few years have done. No. My suggestion would be to calm down, resist the panic and *think*. Art is a discipline. It takes effort and it takes thought. It can take years to master your medium—paints don't do what you want, unless you know them well. Sketching is a hard-won skill and photography a complicated blend of technical and imaginative know-how. Psychotherapy is the same. Like paints, pencils, notes on a score or the strumming on a guitar, psychotherapists have to find a way to work with our medium, we work *with* clients, not *upon* them. We navigate and negotiate; we neither instruct nor demand. So yes, Anthony Storr's[11] observation is true. Psychotherapists are artists. And as Madame X (and James Baldwin) reminded us on that cold, pre-lockdown London night …

Artists are here to disturb the peace. Otherwise, chaos.[12]

References

Conservatives at home. (2020, January 27). *Suella Braverman: People we elect must take back control from people we don't. Who include the judges.* https://www.conservativehome.com/platform/2020/01/suella-braverman-people-we-elect-must-take-back-control-from-people-we-dont-who-include-the-judges.html Downloaded 15 February 2020.

Gilbert, P. (2017). *Depression: The evolution of powerlessness.* Routledge.

Howell, E. (2014). Ferenczi's concept of identification with the aggressor: Understanding dissociative structure with interacting victim and abuser self-states. *The American Journal of Psychoanalysis, 74*(1), 48–59.

Literary Conversations Series. (Undated). *Conversations with James Baldwin,* University Press of Mississippi.

May, R. (1977). *The meaning of anxiety.* Norton and Co. .

---

[11] Storr (1990).
[12] Literary Conversations Series (Undated).

Starkman, H. (2015). Interview with Susie Orbach, PhD, CSW. *Clinical Social Work Journal.* https://doi.org/10.1007/s10615-015-0558-x

Storr, A. (1990). *The art of psychotherapy.* Routledge.

TheyWorkForYou website. (n.d). *Alok Sharma, Minister without Portfolio.* https://www.theyworkforyou.com/mp/24902/alok_sharma/reading_west/votes#environment. Downloaded 21 February 2020.

Thorne, M. (2020). *Getting in good trouble, Remembering John Lewis.* https://www.nasw-michigan.org/news/523810/Getting-in-Good-Trouble.-Remembering-John-Lewis.htm. Downloaded 19 March 2021.

The Reach of Reductionism

In this part contributors look at the way that power plays out through the adoption of reductive and Othering mindsets—with all the advantages and significant problems associated with it. The assumptions that this mindset and its associated concepts—"objective", "dispassionate", "unaffected" by habit and ideology—are inevitably possible or desirable is considered. These ideas underpin, what Naomi Klein calls an extractive mindset, facilitating a way of viewing both the natural world and the majority of its inhabitants. It is a mindset that reduces people, animals and other constituents of the natural world, to resources to use up and discard.[1]

In this part, reductionism is explored in three different areas—academia, our relationship to animals and the political dimension of life.

Helen Damon helps us explore academic life, particularly issues of assessment. She asks us to consider "Objective-ication"—a term she uses to problematise some of the assumptions educators and students have to face. It is a fascinating exploration of what it means when the academy—managers, academics and students alike—reduce people to objects, and

---

[1] Klein (2014).

learning to the demonstration of learning outcomes. Helen's chapter raises questions as to whether this is as useful a clarification as purveyors of this approach suggest it to be and Helen explores the implications of this in detail, drawing on her own experience of academia—both as a student and as faculty.

Dale Judd's autobiographically oriented chapter explores our relationship with other animals, and in particular the place that interpretation has in what has become a contested, contradictory and exploitative relationship. This is an important focus to have because as well as damaging our relationship to other sentient beings, these reductionistic and exploitative approaches are at the heart of the climate and environmental crisis which has damaged—and continues to damage—the planet, the climate and humanity alike. These attitudes impede our efforts to tackle these crises and have been implicated in the spread of novel zoonotic diseases[2] that, as we are currently experiencing, are so catastrophic.

In his chapter Miltos Hadjiosif interrogates the notion of the political—both its discursive and cultural power and the ways in which it affects us personally. In some ways Miltos amplifies questions and concerns from Part I and he is particularly concerned with the fact that the distress people experience (which can bring people to therapy), more often than not, has origins in the social and political. By addressing the fact that the political separates us from one another, and is so destabilising, Miltos takes us full circle and allows us to reconsider the intimate and personal disorientation and distress that is so prevalent.

References

Kenyon, C. (2020). We Need to Address the Underlying Ecological Determinants of COVID-19. *Preprints, 1*, 2020060040. http://doi.org/10.20944/preprints202006.0040.v1.

Klein, N. (2014). *This changes everything: Capitalism vs the climate*. Penguin Books.

---

[2] Kenyon (2020).

"Objective"-ication: Problems with Treating Judgement as Fact

Helen Damon

The phenomenon I call *"objective"-ication* is a perennial source of fascination, power and tension in my life—indeed, as I'll argue, in human life per se. "Objective"-ication—henceforth *objectivication,* for ease of reading—is the phenomenon by which a subjective judgement is taken or treated *as if* it were objective, in the sense of "factual" or "fair", or has consequences that are objective, in the sense of "real". I have chosen to use the terms "objectivication" and "objectivy", rather than "objectification" and "objectify", to emphasise this "as if" quality: the former terms should be used in relation to subjective judgements that are taken or treated *as if* they were objective, whereas the latter terms may also refer to judgements that *are* objective.

As children, we are all subject(ed) to the objectivication of adults' judgements, which is near-absolute and godlike in its scope. At this stage in our lives, even our fundamental bodily needs and functions are controlled, such as whether, what and when we may eat and drink, and

H. Damon (✉)
London, UK

perhaps even whether and when we may go to the toilet. In my childhood, at least, many's the time an officious teacher denied my peers' and my desperate requests to relieve ourselves with the admonishment that "You should have gone at break time: now you'll just have to wait."

As we develop, we come increasingly to recognise that adults' judgements may also be godlike in their arbitrariness and capriciousness—as with the Greco-Roman gods, for example. At primary school, my teachers required me to rule a 2 cm-wide margin in my exercise books. "But my ruler's 2.5 cm wide: couldn't I just –" "No". At secondary school, I was among the first cohort to sit AS Levels, in 2001, and I vividly remember my English teacher announcing that, as no-one yet had a clue what the standard of these newfangled exams might be, she had decided to mark our mocks "as if I were an A-Level marker who'd just had a cup of tea and a biscuit" and was therefore in a particularly generous state of mind. I was aghast at this rude awakening to the partiality and precariousness of the examination system on which the very foundations of my adult life were to be built; aghast at the sheer, agonising farcicality of my prospects riding—rising or crumbling—on a biscuit, and there being nothing, short of stapling a shortbread to my exam paper, I could do about it.

Ultimately, we come to recognise that, much as humans may, indeed, wield godlike power, our capacity for objective judgement is inherently finite and fallible. For example, in jurisdictions that uphold capital punishment, humans wield the power of life and death and, in some cases, have sentenced people to be executed who were innocent of the crimes for which they were convicted. Further, we recognise that "having the capacity to make an objective judgement" and "making an objective judgement" are two different things. God(s) may have the omniscience to make objective judgements yet nonetheless choose to enact a subjective judgement, and mortals may hire their mate over a candidate whom they know has more experience.

As adults, we all almost certainly hold some power of objectivication—as parents, or as members of a hierarchical organisation, for example. As a Lecturer on a professional doctorate in Counselling Psychology, I am acutely aware of holding such power when I mark trainees' assignments. If, in my "professional opinion", I judge that a trainee has "failed" an assignment then, assuming my judgement is upheld by the Examination Board, that trainee must exit the programme. That trainee then fails, in the real, to attain a doctorate and its attendant opportunities. In such moments, I picture myself as if I were a megalomaniacal mythological gatekeeper or videogame final boss, bestride a crossroads, academic robe billowing, mortarboard tassel flailing, barring the way, pronouncing "You shall not pass!" as lightning cleaves the sky. Who am I, who are any of us, to wield such power?

Indeed, the objectivication of my judgements is one of the aspects of my role I find most challenging, philosophically and psychologically. I experience it as a source of cognitive dissonance. In lecturing, I strive to uphold and instil the programme's pluralistic ontology and phenomenological epistemology by encouraging trainees to unpack and challenge the notion that there is (always) one "right answer". However, in marking trainees' assignments, I "must" assess whether they have "given enough of *a* right answer" to pass.

However, pluralism is not relativism, nihilism or anarchy, and "objectivied" judgements are not merely plucked out of thin air—one hopes. Rather, they are most often made in response to one or more shared, external objects that—let's assume, for the sake of argument—exist objectively, even if they are not perceived or appraised (wholly) objectively. Love it or hate it, Marmite exists, objectively, as a food spread made from yeast extract; exhibits are presented as evidence in trials; and, in my work, trainees' assignments are written and evaluated in response to marking criteria.

If you'll forgive my relativisation of an absolute term, I wrote that such external objects may not be perceived or appraised "(wholly) objectively" because, although they are often constructed, they nonetheless often admit of a continuum from the "out-and-out right" to the "out-and-out wrong", and from the "out-and-out objective" to the "out-and-out subjective", within this constructed context. Hence, "having a phobia of cats" and "being allergic to cats" *are* negative characteristics in the context of applying for a job at a cattery, and I defy anyone to argue otherwise. Likewise, every aspect of the assignments I mark is technically a construct, from the arrangement of the shapes "t", "h" and "e" to form "the", and the shared understanding that "the" denotes the "definite article", to the concept of "cognitive behavioural therapy" (CBT). However, an assignment can be more or less close to "rightness"—that is, more or less close to the hypothetical Platonic Form of "the perfect assignment within a given constructed context." For example, within the constructed context of second-wave CBT, "NAT" stands for "Negative Automatic Thought". Fact. It just does, and that's something I know and can therefore assess. Hence, if a trainee writes that it stands for "Neat And Tidy", then they are wrong within this constructed context. Full stop. Conversely, if they write that Aaron Beck, of CBT fame, was born in "1921", then, in the constructed context of the Gregorian calendar, they are right. Fact. Full stop.

However, such conformity to the status quo is one evaluative model among many. One might call it a "Lintottian" model, after the academic approach of the character "Mrs Lintott", a teacher, in Alan Bennett's[1] play, *The History Boys*. If, in completing an assessment, one learns the facts, then reproduces them in a logical, if pedestrian, format, ticking all the boxes of the assessment criteria, then one will pass. "Play up! Play up! And play the game[2]!" Indeed, much of this business of life is a "game"—a constructed activity, with written or unwritten rules, that may be "won" or "lost". Hence, it behoves the referee to play fair by explaining how they interpret the rules, and by following the rules, to give the players a sporting chance. Thus, when setting assignments, I endeavour to explicate, as clearly as possible, how I interpret each marking criterion—to what I frequently worry is a patronising extent. Nonetheless, I'm surprised and exasperated that some trainees in every cohort I've taught so far have taken a bafflingly left-field approach, seemingly wilfully ignoring the criteria. For example, not including therapeutic goals in a CBT assignment when one of the criteria is to do just that.

Perhaps they're playing by different rules—following the "Irwinian" model, after *The History Boys* teacher "Irwin". Irwin asserts that, at Oxbridge, the game is deliberately to get the wrong end of the stick

---

[1] Bennett (2004).
[2] Newboldt (2015).

in order to entertain the assessor. Oxbridge's intention may well be to encourage students to be intellectually playful, challenge dogma and make their own mark in the field. However, as Irwin exemplifies, this, too, can be reduced to a paint-by-numbers performance: a status quo of perverting the status quo; Sartrean bad faith.

It's possible endlessly to debate what a given form of assessment does, and "should", assess. However, the bottom line is that games invite game-playing: to do well in an assessment is to find out what the assessor wants and give it to them, be that conformity, subversion, flattery and so on.

One hopes that, just as judgements aren't plucked out of the air, neither are judges. Just as the "object of judgement"—a CV, an assignment, an action and so on—can be more or less contextually right, so we hold that those who judge possess the ability to identify and evaluate the contextual rightness of such objects to varying degrees. We uphold certain people as "experts" in a given field and seem relatively readily to objectify their "legitimised judgement", wherever on the imagined subjective-to-objective scale it might fall, over others. Want to know if your sourdough's overworked? Ask Paul Hollywood. Want to know if your prose has merit? Contact a literary agent. I presume—at least, I hope—my employer considers me sufficiently qualified to identify and evaluate the contextual rightness of CBT assignments; more qualified, at least, than a layperson. I have, after all, trained in and practised CBT. Certainly, I experience a sense of legitimacy whenever I *am* able to identify the content of an assignment as contextually right or wrong.

We also seem relatively readily to objectify "cumulative subjectives"—that is, multiple concordant opinions—even in the absence of expertise, as in the objectivication of juries' verdicts. However, a critical flaw in this approach is, of course, that two wrongs don't make a right. This approach, to its detriment, does not admit of valid outliers: "[t]hey all laughed at Christopher Columbus/When he said the world was round…", but "[w]ho's got the last laugh now[3]?".

Despite our best efforts to the contrary, human judgement is near-inevitably subject to subjectivity. Take the expert opinion of the judges on the televised dance competition *Strictly Come Dancing*, for example.

---

[3] Astaire and Rogers (1998).

One judge, Bruno Tonioli, scores generously relative to the other three judges: another, Craig Revel Horwood, scores harshly. Yet, both score in proportion to what all the judges seem typically to agree is the overarching quality of the dance. Thus, both give higher scores to "better" dances and lower scores to "worse" dances. However, although a "10" (out of 10) from Revel Horwood is therefore indicative of a higher-quality dance than a 10 from Tonioli, and is therefore "worth more", both "10s" carry the same weight when counted towards a competitor's overall score.

This reminds me of a quotation from Sheila Greenwald's[4] novel, *Will the Real Gertrude Hollings Please Stand Up?*, in which the eponymous heroine, a girl who has been given a diagnosis of Dyslexia, reflects on a jar of dried "Brookwood Black Beans" that her teacher keeps on a bookshelf and uses as reward tokens. She notes that, "…when you see fresh beans at a vegetable store you know that some are fat and some are empty and some are sweeter", but "[j]ust because they're packaged and labelled everyone expects them to be exactly alike[5]". Objectivication, then, perhaps, especially when it stems from quantification, can result in pseudo-homogenisation: a loss of the individual quality of the object(s) of judgement, as here, or of the judgements themselves, as in *Strictly Come Dancing*.

I think we're also inclined to assume that a uniform outcome, such as "These beans are all Brookwoods Black Beans" or "These dances are all 10s", denotes a uniform and perhaps also rational evaluative process, as if the assessor were a—tellingly oxymoronic—"human machine". Yet, I think the "reality", insofar as it exists and can be known, is closest to Kahneman's[6] *two systems* theory of decision-making. According to this theory, we make *system one* rapid, intuitive "gut decisions" by default. However, such decisions derive from a lifetime of introjected experience. Consequently, they are highly likely to be, if not objectively "right", then at least much the same decision as one would have reached via the slower, conscious *system two* process. Thus, the lingerie stylists at *Rigby*

---

[4] Greenwald (1989).
[5] pp. 46–47.
[6] Kahneman (2012).

and Peller have honed the ability to "fit by eye": they are able, accurately, to determine a customer's bra size without recourse to a tape measure. Equivalently, when I read an assignment in a subject I'm familiar with, I have the experience of a mark "popping into my head" that, more often than not, is much the same as the mark I ultimately assign after I've finalised my comments and calibrated all the trainees' marks for a given module against each other.

Why do we seem to strive for—fetishise, even—the quantitative as indicative of a robust and fair judgement, and therefore as legitimising objectivication, especially given how much the objectivity it seems to be taken to denote eludes us? From an existential perspective, it's perhaps symptomatic of a fundamental desire for certainty, consistency and control in the face of a universe that offers anything but. As a striving for fairness, objectivity and the pseudo-objectivity of objectivication are perhaps admirable. However, objectivication might also be perceived as an abdication of responsibility, especially if we conceptualise it as the result of the objective evaluation of something located in the subject of evaluation, rather than primarily as the result of our subjective evaluation of our response to that subject. For example, if we think that "*He is* not good enough for this role" rather than that "*I evaluate him as* not being good enough for this role".

Further, we should be wary of assuming that the objective is necessarily meaningful and valuable, let alone necessarily more meaningful and valuable than the subjective. The objective can be meaningless—or, at least, arbitrary. Van Gogh's *The Starry Night* measures 72 cm x 92 cm, but that's hardly its most meaningful attribute—unless one's tasked with reframing it. Conversely, as anyone who's been on the giving or receiving end of the quintessentially subjective statement "I love you" would attest, the subjective can be profoundly meaningful and valuable.

Although objectivication is problematic, I cannot see how we could avoid it altogether, if only for practical reasons. For example, one could not practicably hire all the candidates who apply for a given job. Thus, any "six of one, half a dozen of the other" attempt at a solution, such as advocating the provision of qualitative descriptions of an assignment's (de)merits, in lieu of a quantitative mark, would not resolve the issue, as long as an objective outcome, such as a determination of a trainee's progression on a course, is required. That said, we can certainly assess what the "best" method of evaluation might be in a given case—although enacting this method would constitute the objectivication of our assessment. Nonetheless, we can endeavour to avoid unnecessary objectivication, such as setting a summative assessment when a formative one would do.

When objectivication is employed, I think "best practice" would essentially entail upholding certain quality criteria common to qualitative research, such as transparency, reflexivity, bracketing and triangulation. If we show, to the best of our ability, how we arrived at a judgement, this will contextualise and demystify it, thus better enabling others to understand and critique it. Such transparency would force us to have, and to be able to articulate, a justification for our judgement, which in turn would force us better to understand and critique our own process. Thus, in marking an assignment, I provide a written commentary on how and to what extent I consider it to meet each marking criterion and on my rationale for awarding it a particular overall mark.

As innumerable psychological studies illustrate, humans rarely make wholly rational, objective and conscious decisions. Rather, our decisions may be impacted by myriad extraneous variables and biases. Consequently, we should endeavour, as far as possible, to identify our positioning in relation to our decisions and to "bracket off" bias. The assignments I mark are not anonymised, and I am mindful that I therefore approach them carrying with me the baggage of my relationship to and expectations of each trainee. At times, I find it difficult to disentangle my assessment of a trainee from my assessment of their assignment. In such cases, I consider it as a best practice to seek a colleague's second opinion. That is, I adopt a triangulated or cumulative subjectives approach, problematic though I've argued that is.

It's also important to be open to our objectivied judgements being discussed, challenged, changed or corrected at any time and by anyone. Lest we forget, it was Toto the dog who exposed the Wizard of Oz as a fraud, and a little boy who denounced the fairytale emperor as wearing no clothes.

Ultimately, I think we should resist the urge to imagine we have shoehorned, or are capable of shoehorning, the square peg of subjectivity into the round hole of objectivity. We should, instead, hold the tension and feel the weight of the responsibility of objectivication. We should remain conscious of and critique it. As such, in a parallel process, I shall endeavour to hold the tension of not having "fixed" the issues raised in this chapter and not having drawn the neatest of tied-with-a-bow conclusions. I've aimed, rather, to raise points and questions of interest in relation to this topic and to encourage reflection and debate. Again in parallel process, I encourage you to critique what I've shown of my working and to draw your own, subjective conclusions about the power and tension of, and possible solutions to, the phenomenon of objectivication where it occurs, be that in teaching, the arts, politics, therapy, parenting or other areas of human experience.

References

Astaire, F., & Rogers, G. (1998). They all laughed [Song]. On *motion picture soundtrack anthology: Fred Astaire and Ginger Rogers at RKO*. Turner Entertainment Co. (Original work published 1937).
Bennett, A. (2004). *The history boys*. Faber and Faber.
Greenwald, S. (1989). *Will the real Gertrude Hollings please stand up?* Puffin Books.
Kahneman, D. (2012). *Thinking, fast and slow*. Penguin.
Newboldt, H. (2015). *Admirals all, and other verses*. Leopold Classic Library.

Animals: Aren't They Great?

Dale Judd

The title of this chapter is deliberately ambivalent and therefore open to *interpretation*. This is my point. It encapsulates perfectly, the paradoxes and ironies which I've come to understand as a white, supposedly "middle-class" (another issue entirely) professional and former meat eater. My main intent in this discussion, is to illustrate how mainstream "Western" society's perception of animals is confused, contradictory and wholly arbitrary, with far-reaching implications for the environment, sustainability and climate change—in fact, the very survival of humanity. While there's a virtual mountain of information and statistical analyses which address the range of environmental effects of eating meat (e.g. land use, water use, habitat destruction, decreasing biodiversity, soil degradation, pollution, deforestation and climate change-inducing CO_2

---

[1] Gibbens (2019).

D. Judd (✉)
Huntingdon, UK

emissions).[1] I won't attempt to repeat it here, although it makes for some grimly fascinating and depressing reading.

The inconsistencies inherent to society's approach can be found everywhere; on any commercial TV channel, you'll see adverts for various meat and fish products, followed by genuinely desperate, emotive appeals from charities such as the Worldwide Fund for Nature (WWF) to help preserve critically endangered species; sausages to snow-leopards within a two minute "ad-break". In a post-modern world with a multiplicity of "truths" it's no surprise then, that a consistent philosophy regarding how we *perceive* and *relate to* our fellow animals hasn't materialised to-date. Taking a wider historical overview, as early religious beliefs formed the basis of "civilised living" (i.e. living within organised social groups) from the polytheists of ancient antiquity to the relatively more recent development of monotheism, the antecedents to this state of affairs in the "modern" world, can be traced back to the bible; Genesis 1:26–28—"mans' dominion over the animals." Although this isn't my main focus, it shows how *interpretations* of the world (and the species within it)—whether through orthodox, religious dogma or biased/selective cultural interpretations, maintains the dissonance inherent to Western society's stance towards animals. Although this discussion concerns the interpretation of animals—in a world of relatedness and inter-dependency, it's ultimately about our interpretations of ourselves.

Interpretation or How to "Make Sense" of the World

It might not seem surprising to learn, that I'm a psychologist by profession, and that therefore, I've been trained to think in certain ways or, that I'm able to consciously "analyse" others and the world around me in order to gain some deeper level of insight or understanding. That would be a perfectly "logical" assumption to make—but it isn't true. If anything, it's the reverse of my experience. I believe that I became a psychologist because I was placed in a position of being an "outsider" early on and always had the sense of looking *in*, instead of feeling that I was "part of the gang".

Being born in a large, industrial market town in central/southern England—Northampton, my family (just myself and my parents) emigrated to the vast expanses of western Canada, to Edmonton, Alberta, in the summer of 1977; I was 6 and a half. Although my memories of first arriving there are vague, what I came to understand as I became older was that I wasn't really *like* the other kids. Although I'm sure most kids feel like misfits at times, which is all part of "growing-up", I had an acute awareness of being dissimilar; I had no connection to Canada, my friends or their families through previous shared experiences, and of course, I was a Brit, as were my parents; my accent soon changed to that of any other Canadian kid, but my parents' didn't. As I became older, these differences began to mean less and I was for all intents and purposes, a Canadian and began to feel comfortable with my new nationality. Ironically, given the focus of this discussion, although I never had any pets other than a goldfish, I was able to experience first-hand, the range of Canadian wildlife (including Grizzly Bears, Moose and Elk) in the National Parks such as Banff and Jasper, in the Rockies of northern Alberta. Unfortunately, the Canadian adventure didn't last; in 1984, when I was 13, nearly 14 in fact, I was told by my parents that we were moving back to the UK! Now this was a problem. At this point, I'm a Canadian teenager and I'd had a Canadian accent for most of my life up to this point. All of my references were North American, although some important things for teenagers, like music and movies were international—everyone listened to the New Romantics of the early 80's and everyone from my generation had watched the original Star Wars trilogy on the big screen. Still, I had no interest in football and no-one in England at this point knew anything about ice-hockey or Wayne Gretzky—you'll need to google him if you don't know. So now I'm back in my "home -town" but feeling more displaced and alien than ever. I had to quickly lose my Canadian accent in order not to stand out, as well as learn a whole new range of slang, local knowledge, TV and entertainment and other cultural references. I also had to wear a school uniform—and there was the weather to get used to as well. Being in my mid-teens with something of a protean identity, this was really the beginning of my understanding of *interpretation* of the world beyond an assumed, *shared* interpretation, which occurs when people are born, raised and remain living within the same place; they might not all like or agree with the same things—but they have a more instant sense of familiarity and connection to the world around them. This wasn't possible for me; I had to *work* at it to try and understand what everyone else took for granted, and where, if at all, I fitted in. So, as you might appreciate, becoming a psychologist for me wasn't a great leap; I'd been consciously doing my own type of "analytical" practice for most of my life.

As a British-Canadian who's had to work at interpreting two different "worlds", for me, the process of *interpretation* is multifaceted and dynamic; it's not simply a set of sensory inputs working together to produce the "outcome", like a Pavlovian, stimulus–response mechanism. It's an active and reciprocal process, that is bound by time, culture, customs, language, beliefs, ideals, prejudices and assumptions. In other words, how we all *interpret* the world around us (including ourselves) is how we *experience* life itself—we give it *meaning*. And, of course, these meanings differ—within cultures, between cultures, family members and so on. The meanings we give to the world through our interpretations, aren't part of a set of universal "truths" but are in essence, the means by which we "make sense" of the world. The branch of philosophy dedicated to this very process is *existential phenomenology*. The main thrust is this—we all have to *interpret* all of our experience of the world throughout life, and therefore, nothing is certain or fixed; life itself is quite literally, meaning*less*. But a note of caution; interpretation in the phenomenological sense, isn't simply a reductive, cognitive process of perception, or a more intellectual process of creating meanings of the world *"out there"*; it has consequences—which are emotional, behavioural, moral, ethical, political, economic or sociological. In other words, we act towards things on the basis of the meanings we give to them.[2] In fact, our interpretations both *create* and *reflect* what we might refer to as "reality". In relation to animals specifically, the consequences are complex and far-reaching.

---

[2] Blumer (1969).

Animal Schisms: To Walk, Wok, Wear, Stroke or Research?

For most of us, especially during childhood, we loved animals, whether through having a pet, watching animal themed TV shows, documentaries, films or even, cartoon animals. As I grew into my teens, like many of my friends at the time, I became more politically conscious and aware of contentious social issues, such as CND, the "Cold War" and others involving animals, particularly vivisection and so-called, blood sports. At some point during the mid to late 1980's, around 1986 to '88, I read an article in a magazine that encouraged readers to write to their local MP, urging them to support a ban on fox-hunting in an upcoming parliamentary debate. It was (and remains) a highly politicised issue. There were often news stories about the efforts of "hunt-saboteurs" clashing with "huntsmen", which I thought was great; these were politically driven outsiders taking on the establishment; this was "class-war". So, with my developing political views and a clearer sense of ethics and morality, I did what any right-minded teen would do—I wrote to my MP. I explained that the outright barbarity of fox-hunting had no place in the late twentieth century; it was simply an anachronism—cruel, vile, hideous. Sometime later, I received a letter from the MP on headed, embossed "Houses of Parliament", heavy weight paper. It was an A5 sheet with a single sentence along the lines of, "whilst *many like yourself feel that fox-hunting is barbaric, I do not believe that government intervention is necessary against this section of society*". I remember vividly, my sense of disappointment and outrage at the time. On a related strand, it's worth including here part of a parliamentary debate from 1993, by the former Labour MP, Tony Banks:

> *There seems to be a close correlation between those who take pleasure in hunting and hurting animals and those who inflict violence on other human beings...Anyone who derives pleasure from the pain and suffering experienced by a fox being hunted by a pack of hounds is on a continuum which, like*

it or not, ends up, in its most extreme form, with the hideous cruelties of a Bosnian massacre or a Nazi death camp.[3]

Personally, I couldn't agree more, although I'm not representing the views of my profession as a British, chartered Counselling Psychologist. The point made by Tony Banks, however, is a powerful one, and well worth considering; all interpretations of reality (however inhumane) become reinforced through social interaction and behaviour.[4] Unfortunately, fox-hunting wasn't banned until The Hunting Act of 2004 which outlawed the hunting of wild mammals with dogs in England and Wales; however, there's overwhelming evidence that the ban is being ignored or exploited by "hunts" on a regular basis.[5]

So, as a teenager, even though I held strong views on fox-hunting in particular, my interpretation of animals at that time, still didn't preclude me from eating meat. I was still able to *selectively interpret* the barbarity and cruelty enacted against *one* species of animal, a fox, while consciously *ignoring* the slaughter of *all farm animals and livestock*. It's a ludicrous and indefensible position to take. Given this inherent dissonance, I have devised an "interpreted conceptual framework of animals", i.e. the ways in which "society" "classifies" animals *through interpretation,* in a *phenomenological* sense, i.e. the *meaning* we attribute to them. The animals in each category aren't intended to be exclusive; they're simply examples of each grouping (Table 1).

These groupings could also be categorised as "animals we like", "animals we use", and "animals trying to survive". However, some of these same animals in the three different groupings are *interchangeable*; our interpretation of animals *isn't* fixed! Thus, one person's pet rabbit can be another's food, a performing dolphin in captivity is clearly part of marine wildlife and an endangered species, such as a tiger, could also be someone else's "exotic" pet. Add to that, the thorny issue of animals *as pet food*—namely, for cats (which are obligate carnivores) and dogs; they both hold a uniquely privileged, interpretative animal status in the

---

[3] House of Commons Hansard Debates (2000).
[4] Berger and Luckmann (1966).
[5] League Against Cruel Sports (2020).

Table 1 Interpreted conceptual framework of animals

Animals for Pleasure	Common' Pets	Cats, dogs, rodents, rabbits, birds, horses, ponies, fish—freshwater or tropical
	Exotic' Pets	Lizard, snakes, spiders, chimpanzees, 'big-cats'
	Preservation/Education	Wildlife parks; Nature reserves; Zoos
Animals for Utility	Food	Livestock'—cows/calves, pigs, sheep, lamb, poultry, fish (wild caught or farmed) rabbits—also horses (France & Italy) and cats & dogs in some parts of the world
	Clothing	Leather is a by-product of the meat industry. Mink, fox, chinchillas, rabbits, and raccoons are 'farmed' for their fur, and cobras, pythons, alligators and crocodiles for their skin. *Each year more than 100 million animals are raised and killed for their fur; 95% is 'farmed'.* (Furfarming, 2020)
	'Working' animals	Guide-dogs, sheep-dogs, police-dogs, police-horses, race-horses, show-jumping horses, donkeys, mules, greyhounds and whippets—(dog racing)
	TV/Film animals	Cats, dogs, horses, bears, 'big-cats', dolphins
	Entertainment (other)	Rodeos (North & South America); 'Sea-World' (USA); Bull-fighting (Spain)
	Research/vivisection	Fish, mice, rats, guinea-pigs, hamsters, rabbits, birds, cats, dogs, mini-pigs, monkeys, chimpanzees. *Estimated - 115 million animals used in laboratory experiments globally each year.* Humane Society International (2021)

(continued)

Table 1 (continued)

	Hunting	Global – different seasons for varied species – big game; safaris in Africa/Asia
	'Blood sports' (Criminal Activity)	Fox-hunting, hare-coursing, badger-baiting, dog-fighting
Animals 'in the wild'	Wildlife	All animals, birds, fish, including larger mammals (Europe/North-America), e.g. bears
	Unwelcome wildlife	'Pests'—e.g. feral rats, pigeons, moles, squirrels, foxes, badgers etc
	Endangered Species	*Total number of globally threatened species* of mammals, birds, reptiles, amphibians and fish as of March 2021= **9914** International Union for Conservation (2021)

N.B. Animals for "entertainment" or "working" animals have been placed under "Animals for Utility" and not "Animals for Pleasure", as their "role" (other than simply needing to be cared for) has been specifically determined for them, which may not be in their best interests

"Western" world. Thus, it appears that we can shift our interpretation, but only when it suits our purposes and, doesn't threaten to seriously challenge our beliefs about ourselves; especially as "animal lovers".

On this issue of the flexibility (or lack of) of our interpretations of animals, I was recently told an anecdote from the world of secondary education; a lesson from a school teacher's GSCE geography class. The lesson was about Sir Ernest Shackleton's disastrous, Antarctic expedition which set off in August 1914, in an attempt to make the first land crossing of the Antarctic.[6] Much like Apollo 13's "Houston we have a problem" just over half a century later, although the expedition failed, it became an epic triumph of survival against all odds. In October 1915, Shackleton's ship, aptly named, *The Endurance*, became trapped and slowly crushed in pack ice just off Antarctica, where it eventually sank, stranding the 28 strong crew, without proper supplies, equipment

---

[6] Lansing (2000).

or, any chance of rescue. In the weeks after they became stranded, Shackleton ordered that the surviving sled-dogs were shot, not just to eat, but because the dogs also required food which they simply didn't have to spare. When the teacher explained these dire circumstances of survival to the students, they were horrified; "But they're *dogs* - you can't just can't shoot them"! In the dichotomous thinking of a secondary school pupil, however, they had no issue at all, with the necessity to kill seals, penguins or other wildlife to survive—but to kill a dog, now that was going too far! This provides a somewhat commonplace (which makes it all the more disturbing) insight into the inherent dissonance in our relationships with animals; it's wholly inconsistent and riven by hypocrisy.

Please bear in mind, however, that I'm *not* suggesting that feral rats would be welcome in your living-room, that the snow-leopard doesn't need our help to be preserved as an endangered species, that your pet cat, dog or hamster, doesn't provide a world of affection and endless fascination, or unfortunately, that millions of Brits don't enjoy eating burgers, sausages, steak, roast chicken—or kebabs. There are seemingly obvious reasons why one would be a pet, another, an endangered species, another a pest, and yet another still, unfortunately, Saturday night's take-away. However, the "elephant in the room" (no pun intended) is that society has determined the very *interpretations* of these animals, and consequently, how we are to *feel* about them which in turn, *dictates* directly, how they are to be *treated* or *used*. This type of "schism" or dissonance in our thinking serves to mask a socially sanctioned indifference and brutality, which through a more considered reflection, is as ludicrous as it is horrific. At one extreme, we have the romanticised interpretation of the pet which is "part of the family", or another, which because of its status as an apex predator (e.g. lions, tigers or bears) is hunted with a high-powered rifle at a considerably safe distance (very "sporting" that) while another still, becomes Sunday's roast. But, if the processes of interpretation create the *meaning*, and the *function* of an animal, how did we come to make these interpretations in the first place?

Meat Is Murder

The Smiths' great, politically strident, second album released in February 1985, "Meat is Murder"; a philosophy captured perfectly in a three-word statement. Morrissey and Johnny Marr (1985) clearly "nailed their colours to the mast" with this one. If you don't know it, the LP's cover image, is a 1967 black and white photograph of a US marine in Vietnam, but slightly altered, with the now iconic phrase written on his helmet. When the album came out, like most others (and by pure mathematics, most readers of this discussion; roughly, only 3% of the UK population are vegetarian)[7] I still ate meat. To this day, the argument remains that we eat meat because we *breed* it specifically for that purpose. Globally, we *slaughter…more than 200 million animals every day—just on land*. That's *72 billion land animals slaughtered globally each year*; if you include wild caught and farmed fish, that's *a daily total closer to 3 billion animals.*[8] That's some very enthusiastic slaughtering. Ironically, many in the UK in particular, would consider themselves as "animal lovers"; as approximately 97% of Brits still eat meat, I find *that* really hard to swallow. The numbers are genuinely shocking and speak for themselves. Although in nature, "big animals eat small animals", as humans, we do of course have a *choice*. Also, the notion of "humane slaughter" must be one of the biggest oxymorons, myths—or just plain lies, which has been around for some time, perpetuated of course by…the meat industry, "hand in glove" with supermarket retail.

And herein, I think, lies the most significant issue regarding how we've come to have this strange, dissonant position on all animal life—most of us *eat* them. But why do we do this? Because like most habitual behaviours, we learned it during early childhood—just like the geography students in the Shackleton lesson above. It's what psychologists or "social scientists" call, *primary socialisation*[9]; how children learn the culturally endorsed interpretations, attitudes, values and behaviour of

---

[7] The Vegetarian Society of the United Kingdom (2020).
[8] Zampa (2018).
[9] Abercrombie et al. (1988).

their culture. If you think of Maslow's hierarchy of needs[10]; if food is one of our most basic needs for survival, and we purposefully *breed* and then *kill* animals for this very purpose, then in our *interpretation* of animals, we've turned them from a creature—a *sentient being*, into a *thing*. It requires an *interpretative shift*, a conscious turning away from an "uncomfortable truth" or more simply—just don't think about it. In fact, it's this very dissonance in our interpretation of animals which is *essential* in order to eat them; we don't kill and eat animals, we're emotionally attached to.

Obviously, meat has to be presented to the shopper in a "consumer-acceptable" way; however, the way in which it's packaged serves a more covert, psychologically significant purpose—to *separate* our interpretation, from the slaughter that was needed to cook shepherd's pie or chicken cacciatore. The aim is to reinforce the interpretation; this is just *food*, not a once sentient creature. Even when I was still eating meat, I always found it strange in a supermarket, looking at the carefully packaged and sanitised pieces of meat, presented as if they had always existed in that strange, plastic-wrapped form, far removed (literally) from the animal from which that leg, thigh, breast or "joint" once belonged. As with the strategies to shock cigarette buyers with the aim of reducing smoking, can you picture the imagery of meat production from abattoirs, positioned above the meat aisle or counter in the supermarket? Of course not, that would be *truly* horrific—as would, the plummeting sales and profits for meat manufacturers. As they say, "no-one likes to see how the sausage is made".

Some readers might be thinking at this point, that I'm presenting some type of left-wing, liberal, bullshit here; "but we're the most *advanced* species on the planet – of course we can breed animals for meat". That's good—it links to the next part of my argument.

---

[10] Maslow (1943).

The War of the Worlds

The classic H.G. Wells novel, *The War of the Worlds*,[11] is set sometime in the first years of the 1900's, and uses a first-person narrative to describe an invasion of Earth by Martians. Due to their advanced, alien technology, the Martians were able to easily over-run any human resistance and proceeded to slaughter humans *en-masse* as a food source, by draining all of the blood from their human victims' bodies. But, because they hadn't evolved to live on Earth, they soon began to die off, through being exposed to microscopic bacteria for which they had no natural defences. It's an inspired and captivating novel, which is widely regarded as the beginning of modern science-fiction. However, on its initial publication in 1898, it was part of a genre of adult fiction known as "invasion literature[12]", reflecting the increasing tensions and insecurities between imperial European powers, which ultimately led to the start of the First World War in 1914. However, Wells' novel didn't appear to be representative of the trope of "invasion anxiety" inspired fiction of its time; *The War of the Worlds* had a far more interesting subtext.

Written at the turn of the twentieth century, although ostensibly, science-fiction, Wells seemed to have been writing a commentary on his closing Victorian era; championing the advances in science, particularly Darwin's Theory of Evolution and Natural Selection,[13] but also, weaving a sly critique about colonialism and Empire.[14] The idea of an advanced, "superior" race being able to easily invade and conquer a far more "inferior" race with impunity, purely because their highly sophisticated technology allowed them to do so, is a brilliant literary analogy; the British Empire was built on this very means.

However, to my mind, it wasn't much of a stretch to view this same process of space-age colonialism, as an analogy about eating meat. The same dynamic of dominance, control and global mass slaughter with regards to animals as food was inescapable. So, with that in mind,

---

[11] Wells and Roberts (2017a).
[12] Wells and Roberts (2017b).
[13] Williamson et al. (2005).
[14] Zebrowski, et al. (2005).

imagine Earth being invaded by aliens who came to discover that humans were actually quite tasty…Mmmm—and then wished to breed *us*, for food! That would be horrific beyond compare—right? Well no, actually it's not. In fact, we're enacting the same type of horror by the very same process, through our own carnivorous behaviours. Remember the figures above—3 billion animals slaughtered globally *per day*! How can it be that our *interpretation* of animals is so *utterly* selective—especially in the UK, as a nation of supposed "animal lovers"? I understand that this will seem ridiculous to some—probably most, with 97% of the population eating meat. But, if you can try and think of this analogy, with humanity as the food source for a "superior" being, I'd hope that it would at least, promote some greater reflection about eating meat, and if it does—great; there's no *need* for any of us to eat meat (including children and pregnant women—NHS)—it's a legacy from our past[15] or, just another learned behaviour.

Conclusions

Hopefully, this phenomenologically informed argument, has provided some "food for thought" on how "Western" society's approach to the whole animal kingdom, is based upon entirely inconsistent, conflicting and arbitrary interpretations of animals, their potential "uses" for humanity and the values which govern our behaviour towards them. My view on this subject is of course, *mine*; it's personal and comprised of different moral, philosophical and environmental strands which collectively have shaped my views and also my behaviour over time i.e. I'm a vegetarian. But, if anyone has taken exception to anything discussed here, then I'd welcome it; it's only through expressing differences of opinion that hopefully, an informed dialogue can be created, and through which other possible interpretations, meanings and understandings can be generated. In an increasingly divisive world, what's needed is more dialogue, not less.

---

[15] NHS (2018a, 2018b).

Although this discussion concerned society's conflicting interpretations of animals, it was simultaneously, about our interpretation of ourselves. As *homo sapiens,* we are without doubt, the most dominant (and *wilfully* destructive) species on the planet; a parasite in fact. This is ironic, given that homo sapiens is Latin, for *wise man.* Unfortunately, it seems that through this dominance, the arrogance and complacency that accompanies it, and our preoccupations with material goods and increasing personal wealth, that we've also forgotten something very fundamental; we are *dependent upon* and *defined by* our co-existence with the planet and, to the millions of other species that we *share* with it. Hence, for the existentialists, human existence (or *Dasein* in the original German) is literally, "*being-in-the-world*[16]". So, if humanity is to survive much beyond the twenty-first century, and we're to act like a responsible "custodian" of the planet and its species, we need to keep one thing in mind; although we need the Earth, it certainly doesn't need us—it will be here long after humanity has disappeared. It's one of the things that I find completely disingenuous about the environmental movement; the talk of "saving the planet" is actually, nothing of the sort—it's about saving humanity. Perhaps if the message was changed, the *interpretation* would change with it, and the climate change deniers might pay more attention to the plight of humanity?

And so then, what is the answer? While there are certainly other possible interpretations available to us, unfortunately, what appears to be lacking the most, is the necessary personal motivation, or political will, from those "in charge". We have insight, but as is often the case, it isn't enough to change behaviour. For instance, there's absolutely no need for any school meals in the UK to include meat; but perhaps that message needs the support of a celebrity, TV chef? Early socialisation with *not* eating meat would be a fundamental step—not only to slow the slaughter, but ultimately, to reinforce the interpretation that we *don't* eat animals and in so doing, help to give humanity a much-needed lifeline.

Any process of change has to start somewhere and so why not with yourself? I hope that having discussed the arbitrary, inconsistent and hypocritical stance that we adopt through our interpretations of animals,

---

[16] Heidegger et al. (1962).

you'll begin to reconsider your own and stop eating them—or less often to start with. From my own experience, once I was able to challenge myself and remove the all too cosy confines of my previously un-reflected interpretations and assumptions, it was surprisingly easy. Remember; we do have a choice—both in our interpretations *and* in our behaviour.

On this issue of *choice*, on the edge of Hyde Park in London, is *The Animals in War Memorial*, a striking monument constructed in Portland stone and bronze; the memorial has two inscriptions:

> "This monument is dedicated to all the animals that served and died alongside British and Allied forces in wars and campaigns throughout time".
> "They had no choice[17]".

A simple and sombre statement of fact; a fitting conclusion to this discussion. Equally, there could be a companion-piece memorial for the world's animals slaughtered for meat, fur or skin, who also had (and continue to have) no choice. In our globally consumerist world, the most significant power any of us have is this; *the choice of what we spend our money on*. Just imagine if those UK statistics were reversed; 97% of the population were vegetarian and only 3% ate meat; that would be the result of an entirely different, *interpreted world*; nothing less in fact, than a process of *conscious (r)evolution*; so, what's *your* interpretation of animals now?

References

Abercrombie, N., Hill, S., & Turner, B. S. (1988). *The penguin dictionary of sociology* (p.231). Penguin Books.

AIW. (2020). *The animals in war memorial.* http://www.animalsinwar.org.uk/. Retrieved 1 March 2020.

Berger, P. L., & Luckmann, T. (1966). *The social construction of reality: A treatise in the sociology of knowledge*. Penguin Books.

Blumer, H. (1969). *Symbolic interactionism: Perspective and method*. Prentice-Hall.

---

[17] AIW (2000).

Fur Free Alliance. (n.d.). *Fur farming.* https://www.furfreealliance.com/fur-farming/. Retrieved 6 January 2020.

Gibbens, S. (2019, January 17). Eating meat has 'dire' consequences for the planet. *National Geographic.* https://www.nationalgeographic.co.uk/environment-and-conservation/2019/01/eating-meat-has-dire-consequences-planet-claims-british-report. Retrieved 6 January 2020.

Heidegger, M., Macquarrie, J., & Robinson, E. (1962). *Being and time.* Harper & Row.

Holy Bible: King James Version, Genesis 1:26–28. Collins.

House of Commons Hansard Debates for 27 April 1993. (2000). https://publications.parliament.uk/pa/cm199293/cmhansrd/1993-04-27/Debate-1.html. Retrieved 4 February 2020.

Humane Society International. (2021, October 21). *About animal testing.* https://www.hsi.org/news-media/about/. Retrieved 12 January 2020.

International Union for Conservation (IUCN). (2021). *The IUCN Red List of Threatened Species.* Version 2020–3. https://www.iucnredlist.org. Retrieved 30 January 2021.

League Against Cruel Sports. (n.d.). *Fox hunting.* https://www.league.org.uk/fox-hunting. Retrieved 4 February 2020.

Lansing, A. (2000). *Endurance: Shackleton's incredible voyage to the Antarctic.* Weidenfeld & Nicholson.

Maslow, A. (1943). A theory of human motivation. *Psychological Review, 50*(4), 370–396. https://doi.org/10.1037/h0054346.

Morrissey, S., & Marr, J. (1985). *The Smiths: Meat Is Murder [LP].* Warner Music.

NHS. (2018a). *Vegetarian and vegan mums-to-be.* https://www.nhs.uk/live-well/eat-well/vegetarian-and-vegan-mums-to-be/. Retrieved 17 February 2020.

NHS. (2018b). *The vegetarian diet.* https://www.nhs.uk/live-well/eat-well/the-vegetarian-diet/. Retrieved 17 February 2020.

The Vegetarian Society. (2020). *Facts and figures.* https://vegsoc.org/info-hub/facts-and-figures/. Retrieved 13 January 2020.

Wells, H., & Roberts, A. (2017a). Introduction. *The war of the worlds* (pp. 9–15). Gollancz.

Wells, H., & Roberts, A. (2017b). *The war of the worlds.* Gollancz.

Williamson, J., Yeffeth, G., & Wells, H. (2005). *The war of the worlds: Fresh perspectives on the H. G. Wells classic* (pp. 189–195). BenBella Books.

Zampa, M. (2018, September 16). *How many animals are killed for food every day?* https://sentientmedia.org/how-many-animals-are-killed-for-food-every-day/. Retrieved 6 January 2020.

Zebrowski, G., Yeffeth, G., & Wells, H. (2005). *The war of the worlds: Fresh perspectives on the H. G. Wells classic* (pp. 235–241). BenBella Books.

Balancing on Quicksand: Making Sense of What "The Personal is Political" Means

Miltos Hadjiosif

Prologue

We are in the world of "Game of Thrones". It is Season 1, the episode where Jorah Mormont explains to Daenerys that the Dothraki have a right to rape and pillage the flock of lambs-people they have just conquered. Daenerys looks upon the unfolding horror mortified, and as she takes in the pain, spurs to action in what is one of the first instances of her exercising her recently acquired power: that of Queen, or to be more precise, *Khaleesi*. She peels a Dothraki warrior off a woman and claims her as a handmaiden. The warrior begrudgingly complies. Sir Jorah, her protector, gently offers: "you cannot claim them all *Khaleesi*". And as the mesmerising word for Dothraki Queen materialises in sound through his impeccable accent, she replies: "I can. And I will."

M. Hadjiosif (✉)
Bristol, UK
e-mail: miltos.hadjiosif@uwe.ac.uk

© The Author(s), under exclusive license to Springer Nature Switzerland AG 2021
M. Milton (ed.), *Balancing on Quicksand*,
https://doi.org/10.1007/978-3-030-79136-0_7

This defiant phrase comes to mind as I am confronted with the many entangling issues invoked by "politics and psychotherapy". I am joking; I can't claim or speak to all these issues. I need to start with humour, else I will drown. I have succumbed to the darkness that lies both inside and all around me before. A familiar terror thus returns, compelling me to stand still. I know what it feels like to be trying to balance on quicksand. Give me strength *Khaleesi*. You deserved a better ending…

A Glimpse from Athens in the 90s

I remember reading that "the personal is political" for the first time. It kind of made sense, but not really. The phrase has its origins in second-wave feminism,[1] when it was used as a slogan by consciousness raising groups to alert women that the violence and domestic struggles they experienced where rooted in patriarchy and other systems of oppression; thus liberation entailed a form of collectivisation as opposed to individual solutions for solitary predicaments. I came of age in 90s Greece, a setting that was hardly conducive to making the link between personal experience and politics. Despite converting to social constructionism during my undergraduate studies in psychology, quite what this statement signified still eluded me. Counselling psychology training should, in theory, make it blatantly clear that the distress one encounters in the consulting room, more often than not, has origins that are well beyond its remit. While in training, we had some exposure to systemic therapy, which terrified us at the time, as it generated questions that could potentially derail our trust in our "empathic listening skills". For example, what is the point of working with the aftermath of domestic violence if our profession is unable to tackle its origins? Where are the perpetrators; shouldn't they be in therapy instead of their partners? How can we help young clients navigate increasingly competitive and toxic environments that breed so much incongruence? Indian philosopher Jiddu Krishnamurti is said to have noted "It is no measure of health to be well adjusted to a profoundly sick society", but it is Eddie Vedder (the lead singer of

---

[1] Mackay (2015).

Pearl Jam) who expressed a variant of this that led me to embrace it as a moral philosophy. I am slowly realising just how political grunge music was, and how it alerted us to the tapestry of social ills that its protagonists plotted in their lyrics. Hardly anyone argued back then that grunge is a gateway to political consciousness raising. Or maybe they did, and I wasn't paying attention. In a world that has been declared post-modern yet feels increasingly regressive, one cannot look to a single place or starting point to begin the journey of understanding how exactly the personal is political.

If I could speak to my pre-pubescent self, I would tell him something which might seem obvious today: politics is not synonymous with "party politics" and even though you might not be into it, it certainly is into you. I look back to ordinary and recurring scenes of Athenian civic life, such as when a holiday was celebrated among family and friends and the men would sit in the living room arguing about politics while women prepared food in the kitchen while exchanging vacuous pleasantries. If I could go back, I would go up to them, all of them, and in my signature precocious style shout: "Stop talking about politics; you are *doing* politics". I might have been tempted to list their marital strains, which somehow where pretty obvious to all us kids, and tell them to sort them out and finish with a group hug. But of course, my pre-pubescent self would understand none of this and a painful truth hits me again. You don't raise awareness like this. For systemic change to occur, you need to engage hearts and minds. "I've seen the error of my ways and will own my projections" said nobody ever in response to a 9-year-old's tantrum. Collective action is just that, collective. "But if everyone wants to be a leader, who will be left to follow?" At least I was able to think that in response to the stupid "be a leader, not a follower" messages MTV was feeding us in between some terrific music videos.

The Personal Becomes Political

Coming out as a gay man was one of the most difficult challenges of my adult life. Growing up in Greece, I unwittingly absorbed and embodied every ounce of homophobia that my proud countrymen served me as a child: from the outright toxicity of the "aberration" discourse down to the dollops of derision and judgement couched in jokes and stereotypes of what gay men are supposed to sound like, look like, and act like. For various reasons, it wasn't until my mid 20s that I rode a life-affirming wave of congruence nurtured by my training, to announce to my entire circle of family and friends, in the space of 2 weeks, that I was gay. Their reactions were as good as I could have realistically expected, and everyone declared their support in one way or another. I accurately predicted that dad would quench his feelings with well-intentioned but inauthentic reassurance, whereas mum would freak out initially, thus processing, and ultimately arriving at acceptance, quicker. The advantage of coming out while equipped with some life-wisdom and psychotherapy training is that one is perhaps less vulnerable to the inescapable awkwardness involved and can do so while remaining experience-near. In short, I knew intuitively that for the people that mattered, I had to allow them some time to process and ask questions that needed to be asked.

I did not initially experience my coming out as a political act. That is until a few months later, while sitting on my best friend's balcony, which has always been somewhat of a sanctuary for me. We were enjoying a casual spring evening with a small group of friends. My recollection is that there was lightness in the air and laughter came easy. Present in that encounter was a young woman who I did not know very well; she was spirited and rather nosy in a benign way. At some point she told me that she wanted to find out more about gay relationships and gay sex. She asked a series of progressively clumsier questions and when this culminated in: "do you take the role of woman or man in the relationship?", time froze, and I could sense my heterosexual friends getting ready to jump at her. I remember the feelings I felt. Anger, shame, and the creeping sense that there aren't many ways to steer this conversation in a mutually beneficial direction. But it dawned on me there and then for the first time that, while I could shut this question down, I could also do something else. I looked at her and slipped into my therapist self: "I wonder what drives this question?" I offered in an attempt to buy time and process the next response. What I experienced was someone genuinely, albeit naively, curious to find out something about the "other". There was no judgement, no specific answer she was looking for, no intent to hurt me as far as I could tell. I answered her question in a way that I don't recall, which almost certainly involved the word "deconstruction". She must have registered that she touched a nerve, asked for my permission and kept quizzing me, my answers filling her with delight and fuelling further questions. Someone in the group, eventually said to her: "ok, your turn to tell us how you like your cock". Overall, a pleasant evening.

More than 10 years have passed since this evening. For a long while, I relished this encounter because it captures something about the "offence culture" that we are currently immersed in. I felt pride in not taking offence. If a gay man does not accept some responsibility for showing others what it means for him to be a gay man, how on earth is the ignorant "other" meant to find out? I believe these self-congratulatory thoughts miss a point, however. It should not be left to marginalised and oppressed minorities to do the hard work of consciousness raising and educating ignorance. Psychotherapy training should most certainly not be a pre-requisite to navigate and endure the excruciating death by a thousand cuts involved in what has come to be known as "microaggressions". The tremendous amount of support and meticulous planning I had at my disposal, amplified by my social capital, allowed me to seek and co-construct an experience that fused the personal with the political; a choice if you like that grew out of this intersection. The encounter can only be rendered meaningful against a backdrop of hard-won civil rights and destigmatising policies for the LGBTQ community. Going back in time, "offence" and its derivative affective component, rage, were necessary to enact legislative agendas whose aftermath offered me a position to speak from, and later inhabit more fully, as I grew into an understanding of this issue as both a private and a public matter. Rage, laced with hope, is what I feel as I support the global "Black Lives Matter" (BLM) protests ignited by the summer 2020 events. Rage only towards any utterance of the absurd "All Lives Matter". Gross. Yet, even as my face contorts into disgust while writing this, I have a niggling suspicion that the phrase carries different meanings and cannot simply be shot down. My whiteness, its particular shade (i.e. the Cypriot "off-white" variety), and how it joins the BLM movement is a work in progress.

So how can we resolve this tension? How does one witness and validate the rage, collective and individual, without splitting the world into binary categories of "good" and "bad", when language emerges variably as a tool of toxicity, ignorance, policing or virtue signalling? And how did we end up in a discussion on diversity? I believe the answer to the last question is relatively straightforward. Talking about politics in the twenty-first century means taking stock of multiple heretofore muted voices. As previously silenced groups of people are gaining visibility and attempt to participate in civic life, their needs come into focus, and practices that used to conserve a multitude of "-isms" are called into question.

On the contrary, providing an answer to the first question only invites more questions, and no position feels unassailable. "Social justice warrior" is an accusation that has been both levelled at me and one I have ascribed to others. "Doer" and "done to", as Jessica Benjamin would say, are positions that I occupy intermittently, and neither feels comfortable or lasts too long, as I see both privilege and oppression intersecting. I suspect that resolution might be the wrong way to think about this. I realise that asking "how do we resolve this" is a flawed question. It's "how do I balance this". Really, this is a personal quest that involves a degree of willingness to listen, to argue, to apologise, to get it really wrong, to bear guilt and bear witness. "Extinction Rebellion" believes that shaming people does not make them change, and I have heeded this advice as I notice the almost sadistic pleasure I get from shaming older family members too cushy to act on the concerns of the "snowflake generation". Blinding moral certainty, it turns out, is usually met by negation. Cue "cancel culture".

In trying to achieve a balance of political activism, connectedness and wellbeing, I avoid social media as I can't cope with the barrage of information and the dizzying spins of the news cycle. I sink further into quicksand when I see snippets of decontextualized rhetoric bounce off the echo chamber that many of our social media accounts have become. I believe we need lived experience narrated, nuanced and responded to in prosaic contexts (think town assembly rather than academic paper) in addition to a policy framework that will entrench civil rights into law. However, policy alone is not going to win over any hearts and is likely to be experienced as censorship by some. Hearts and minds. A balance of sorts, even as these two words obscure the bodies that house both and suffer from each.

The Neo-liberal Subject

As critical scholarship has matured through interdisciplinary dialogue, what has been called "neo-liberal subjectivity" has come into sharp focus. I was drawn to the term "subject" during my undergraduate studies in psychology. Broadly speaking, this term is favoured by psychologists who reject alternatives such as "self" and "personality" because they denote something both internal and more or less static; that is, they are essentialisms. We talk about our "self" and "personality" as if they are real, discoverable, and acted upon by our experiences, genes, parenting and so on. Another alternative, "identity", has recently been mired in the semantics of the culture wars and, despite social psychologists' proclamations as to its fluidity, it appears like anything but from a public discourse perspective. The term "subject" allows for the consideration of agency and subjugation alike and speaks to a more abstract "seat of selfhood" as well as the very complex interaction (if we can even call it that) between private and public spheres. I guess, for me, it captured something about my experience of going through life. How did I become a subject? How do I regulate myself according to, or against, ideological imperatives, discourses and the positions my life afforded and denied me? What happens to me when I collide with other subjects?

These questions take me back to my last two years of high school, when I attended a prestigious private school, after persuading my parents to stretch their finances to fund my place. I think this is an important detail for the discussion at hand, as I was not *sent* to that school; I chose it after hearing about its innovative (for the time) provision of the International Baccalaureate (IB) curriculum. My experience of this school was positive in many ways. For the first time in my life I really enjoyed class time, courtesy of some top notch teaching. I managed to make new friends, mostly with other pupils who came from "outsider schools" and existed outside the hierarchy of the native elites. I asserted my independence and signalled my disassociation from them by refusing the school bus and using public transport. Shockingly, for someone so desperate to belong and appear popular and "normal", I was not at all concerned with being accepted by the "in-group" of the rich and powerful Athenian progeny. I found myself in teachers' good graces effortlessly and was strongly encouraged to apply to Oxbridge. Another site of resistance then, as I determined to go to Edinburgh, which was an "alternative" choice under those circumstances.

Attending that school offered me enormous privilege in the form of social capital. Even though I rejected most of its rituals and signifiers, it shaped me by dis-association as I sought to define myself as "not that". I learned to wear my socioeconomic status as a badge of honour, yet soon discovered that the chasm I experienced from the majority of my classmates was dwarfed by the one between me and people from truly disadvantaged backgrounds. Despite my rebellious acts of self-determination, attending that school impacted me in ways I did not foresee. We were reared on a diet of ambition and entitlement as we became globalised almost overnight; our sights now set on the world stage, which instantly rendered ties to our grandparents' villages,[2] a quaint detail to be shared at cocktail parties rather than a meaningful link to our country's history and geography. Greece suddenly became too small for newly acquired, or amplified, ambitions; something that was not helped by the fact that the IB qualification is not recognised by Greek universities. The psychological paradox created by this absurdity is hard to overstate. If your "elite" education offers a route to Harvard but not the Aristotle University of Thessaloniki, one is bound to conclude that either the former (IB) or the latter (Greek universities) are "not good enough". Guess which one was implicitly positioned as inferior in our emerging academic sensibilities. Now you might imagine how that sentiment takes root when a 16-year-old is confronted by Greeks who hold the opposing view. More contradictions and psychological entanglements. The stellar curriculum belied a system that valued competition

---

[2] Few Greeks of my Grandparents' generation hail from Athens, which was only urbanized in the mid-20th Century.

rather than solidarity, intellect over feeling, performance in lieu of experience and money rather than compassion as the standard of worth. At the end of each term, we were ranked according to our exam scores. I pretended I didn't care and condemned the practice, but secretly I was pleased with my performance. Unbeknownst to us, we were being prepared for an envied life and the pursuit of a string of accolades that would help us walk through doors already opened with the reassurance that we did it ourselves. When your entry into adulthood is stamped with the implicit message that life is a CV building activity, then it's hard to pause and take stock of the favourable conditions that created the bullet points on that resumé.

I cannot tell you exactly when I stepped out of that path, other than it was the adversities in my own life that led me to fall and pause (unwillingly) and then bide my time while recalibrating (willingly) before I stood back up. I can also say that connecting my private suffering with structural and systemic matters came with feelings of doubt and guilt. Blaming the "system" for one's experiences often blurs with newfound political awareness and poses challenges to the capacity to take responsibility. As my reflections escaped the narrow confines of that one particular school, I was able to connect with and take interest in issues such as access to healthcare, education policy, workers' rights, the inclusivity agenda, housing and mental health, history (both local and global), and above all, the psychological echoes of neo-liberalism. This term was key for me; it made politics intelligible and penetrable as I recognised it in my schooling experience. I shall not attempt to define it; I would rather tell you how I experience it: as a feeling of "dis-connectedness", not overwhelming, but enduringly underlying. It is simmering under the exchange of ego-inflating remarks, bubbling away at the fringes of consumerism, warping relationships into social status goals. It's a refusal to engage with ideology simply because it worked in your favour, or even if it didn't, this just proves how "hard work and determination" are the only ingredients for success. In a nutshell: quicksand. Whereby the only means of escape is to let it crush you a little bit before you figure out how to emerge, and where to seek more stable footing. Well, this sums it up for me at least.

The connections to mental health are, perhaps, already apparent. So-called mental health issues proliferate in any environment laced with neo-liberal values as distress can only find expression within a limited repertoire of causal explanations: bereavement; a diagnosis assumed to have a biochemical or genetic basis; difficult upbringing. In short, nothing that spells out the broader conditions under which people relate to other people. It is very well established that poverty in the context of inequality, as well as various forms of exclusion and/or oppression, is causally related to people becoming psychologically unwell. What is not as well documented is how people coming from socially privileged and financially comfortable backgrounds become[3] unwell. Looking at the manifestation of severe distress among the so-called "worried well", binding threads can be discerned between the relentless pursuit of happiness, the productivity imperative, the transactional nature of interpersonal relationships and the dominance of cognitivism as an explanatory model of human activity. The common denominator can be described as the interplay between the cult of the (competitive) individual and growth for the sake of growth, which sounds scarily similar to the ideology of cancer, if there ever was such a thing. The neo-liberal subject is simply not compatible with, or at least makes life very challenging for, the relational subject.

Thus, "the personal is political" invites a contextual examination of people's distress and an attention to neo-liberal subjectivity, the spaces it carves out, and what happens to those that for one reason or another are marginalised from participating in its institutions and claiming a "normal" life in its name. As a lecturer in Counselling Psychology working in a British university, I witness first-hand, the pull our students feel towards an auditable surface that coheres around their most marketable correlates. And while they retreat into polished avatars of themselves, we talk about the student mental health crisis as if it can be located and acted upon within their heads. Perhaps some symptoms can, yet its

---

[3] Notice how the verb *become* implies a previous state of health and legitimises the search for a cause that disrupted it. Such is the trickery of language and the caution we must exercise in articulating "truths" about human psychology. Quicksand strikes again.

roots are festering in the nooks and crannies of spaces between them, as they struggle to connect in the age of information and the predations of "surveillance capitalism[4]".

Politics in and from the Consulting Room

Perhaps the greatest sin psychotherapists have collectively committed over the last 100 years is how they have offered *psy* knowledge to the altar of rationality; we too are guilty of making people believe that the world and its people can be reduced to something that is completely fixable, predictable, and controllable. Thus, when one practices psychotherapy influenced by the notion that the personal is political, a number of implications, or rather possibilities, emerge: the first one being a deep suspicion of the neo-liberal objective to appear normal and make sense. The extent to which the issues sketched above can be thought about and worked with in the consulting room is a function of both idiosyncrasy and the constraints within which one is practicing. In other words, attempting to extract "practitioner points" (as some journals are so fond of doing) from this conversation amounts to a dumbing down of the issues and robs the practitioner of the wisdom that can only be gleaned through grappling with them.

Since my training days, I have struggled to envision one-to-one work as aligned with a social justice agenda and psychotherapy as a personal and collective liberation project. I have wondered for years whether "equality is the best therapy".[5] My journey has brought me into contact with people who have felt this struggle, the emotional succour that accompanied such interactions acting as both a vital pre-requisite for my own well-being and a reminder of the power of collective action. I remember a senior therapist at a conference, who shared that she is too old to engage in grassroots activism yet contributes to the causes she

---

[4] Zuboff (2019).

[5] This is one of the slogans that Psychologists for Social Change (previously Psychologists against Austerity) have used.

believes in by offering free psychotherapy to activists, so that they can do their "street work more safely, more fulfillingly".

As psychotherapy is changing with the times, our practices under its remit can illuminate the social and material conditions that our clients are embedded in without sacrificing the depth of subjective experience or the rich messiness of narrative accounts. We now have at our disposal resources that seriously challenge psychiatric diagnoses as they shift attention to issues like power and subjectivity.[6] Central to this deconstruction, in my view, is dismantling the idea that being "client-centred" is equivalent to slavish attachment to articulated client "goals" when therapy begins, such as for instance, when people seek help in order to simply "feel better" or "achieve more" or become comfortable with their own oppression.

Therapy can become a vehicle through which the psychologization of social problems (such as an unemployment) occurs. IAPT (Improved Access to Psychological Therapies[7]) was an economist-conceived initiative to roll out therapy to as many people as possible and was driven by a declaration of mental health as Britain's biggest social problem. The idea was that we needed to get help to those who are unemployed and unproductive so that they can re-enter the workforce and reduce the strain on the public purse. This created thousands of new jobs for psychology graduates, who were seen as the primary population that would staff such a large-scale program. Practitioner psychologists were seen as too expensive to deliver brief, "low intensity" interventions, and were intended to manage the emerging services, organise the referral pathways and supervise those working at the frontline. With that in mind, we can turn our attention to the consulting room itself and understand it as an already politicised space, to which people arrive with certain narratives about themselves, as they offer up their "anxiety" and "depression" for therapeutic intervention.

The NHS, an institution where many of us trained and hold in such high regard, remains a cumbersome medical setting. Precious session time is devoted to administrative tasks, which proliferate under a system

---

[6] Johnstone et al. (2018), Parker et al. (1995), and Watson (2019).
[7] See Layard (2005).

of managed care such as the one envisioned by IAPT. In private work, there is pressure on professionals to compete in a saturated marketplace fraught with blurring professional identities. As therapists' online profiles seek to accentuate their skills by making reference to the brands of therapy they are trained in, so do clients come somewhat primed to try this product out. Thus, theoretical diversity is understood in commercial terms and therapy as psychosocial healing practice becomes less tenable as an aspiration and downright impossible to justify on an insurance form claim. Goodman[8] speaks of this situation as the McDonaldization of psychotherapy, likening manualised therapies to processed food, both devoid of nutrients but nonetheless appealing to consumers and policy makers alike. It is this McDonaldization that I believe we can most insistently name, resist and offer alternatives to. Drawing a parallel between jazz freestyle and a community psychology approach, Nina Browne writes:

> I'm a clinical psychologist by training. It's 'classical' in that you're taught a traditional method of playing, based on some core theories and ideas. But in order to change policy, you have to improvise with the knowledge base. Everyone requires highly fluid roles, a departure from the music sheet. A different audience need the notes in new ways, with space for others to start improvising with you.[9]

The consulting room, symbolically speaking now, is also a space from which to comment on what is happening in the world. It is from a psychotherapeutic perspective that I have come to understand climate change denial as a form of narcissism[10] that denies our most important dependency: our planet and its ecosystems. Similarly, the politics of hate delivered upon narratives of change and a return to glories past (both notable features of the last two US elections and the Brexit campaign) are captured in the notion of splitting and the resultant need to locate the

---

[8] Goodman (2016).
[9] Browne (2019, p. 2).
[10] Lack of empathy and grandiosity are more commonly included in lay descriptions of narcissistic pathology; when arguably of equal importance is the disavowal of the vulnerability that comes with feeling dependent on others.

source of all grievance in a nominal "bad object". I see the relationship between politics and psychotherapy as bidirectional in that both stand to be illuminated by making reference to the other.

Epilogue

A pause here. Politics and Psychotherapy. What a headfuck; where to begin, how to conclude? I attempted to mine my personal history in order to illuminate significant moments that have scaffolded my understanding of the political dimension of my vocation. I hope I have *failed better*[11] than last time at connecting the personal with the social, as I admit to still finding profound meaning in a profession that is currently pondering whether psychologists should seek prescription rights for drugs, with no reference whatsoever to the political implications of such a move. Looking back at my journey, which is still ongoing, and has a relational orientation in lieu of destination, I can describe it as a series of important pivots. I am happy to report that songs, such as the opening track of Skunk Anansie's sublime second album, were just as important as books and conferences, but not as important as the other people I encountered on my way. Even though opening the doors to politics has, at times, literally felt like drowning in quicksand, now that I have felt its texture against my skin, I'm not afraid of it as much. I have cultivated empathy for people who say: "it's too much, I can't think of this right now", where previously I would have either sought to annihilate them with self-righteous indignation or invite them to join me in my quicksand so that we can drown blissfully enmeshed, depending on which phase of my life we're talking about.

Another pause as the second wind escapes my fingers and blows crumbs off the keyboard. A true pause this time… My imagination summons Daenerys again to paraphrase her: "Perhaps I cannot make [therapy] good, she told herself, but I should at least try to make [it] a little less bad." I lied to you earlier when I said that I would try to explain what "the personal is political" means. I didn't know it at the

---

[11] Prall (2004).

time though. I'm still trying to figure it out and it's probably the case that you also need to figure it out for yourself. *Valar politicalis.*

Acknowledgements My gratitude goes to Christine, Derya and Martin who provided helpful comments on earlier drafts of this chapter. And to Giannis and Eftihia for that balcony on Menippou Street.

References

Browne, N. (2019). Don't fear jazz. *The Psychologist, 32*, 2.
Goodman, D. M. (2016). The McDonaldization of psychotherapy: Processed foods, processed therapies, and economic class. *Theory & Psychology, 26*(1), 77–95.
Johnstone, L. & Boyle, M. with Cromby, J., Dillon, J., Harper, D., Kinderman, P., Longden, E., Pilgrim, D., & Read, J. (2018). *The power threat meaning framework: Towards the identification of patterns in emotional distress, unusual experiences and troubled or troubling behaviour, as an alternative to functional psychiatric diagnosis.* British Psychological Society.
Layard, R. (2005). Mental health: Britain's biggest social problem? *LSE Strategy Unit Seminar on Mental Health.* http://eprints.lse.ac.uk/47428/. Retrieved on 6 October 2020.
Mackay, F. (2015). *Radical feminism: Feminist activism in movement.* Palgrave.
Parker, I., Georgaca, E., Harper, D., McLaughlin, T., & Stowell-Smith, M. (1995). *Deconstructing psychopathology.* Sage.
Prall, W. (2004). Failing better: Integrative theory as work in progress. *British Journal of Psychotherapy Integration, 1*(1), 24–32.
Watson, J. (Ed.). (2019). *Drop the disorder! Challenging the culture of psychiatric diagnosis.* PCCS Books.
Zuboff, S. (2019). *The age of surveillance capitalism: The fight for a human future at the new frontier of power.* Profile Books.

Judgement, Discrimination and Stigma

The navigation of social relations often takes us into sticky terrain. Like Schopenhauer's Porcupine we are in a constant dynamic, pulled between the need for closeness on the one hand and the desire for independence on the other. It's a process in which we assess, judge and act towards people—not just as individuals in their own right, but as members or representatives of a group. This isn't totally problematic, in fact at times it is helpful. But difficulties arise when these groupings are too strongly held and stereotyping reigns. When that happens we see assumptions of sameness and difference, fuelling experiences of arbitrary and forced in-groups or out-groups. Alongside this interpretive process, power is used to divide and conquer, to benefit those of the in-group to the detriment of the out-group.

While we see a great deal of division at the moment, we are also seeing alternative, more inclusionary movements that challenge splitting and discrimination. With Black Lives Matter, #MeToo and annual Pride marches, racism and white supremacy are very much under the spotlight, as is misogyny, homophobia and transphobia and other insidious discriminations. We are grappling with the tension of recognising distinct experiences, as well as shared experiences of oppression. Allies are proving to be very important.

This is important as it is not only clear cut "bad guys"—overt racists, transphobes or misogynists—who make assumptions and judge, it is a part of humanity's cognitive armoury, individually and systemically. Even anti-racists exist in—and benefit from—systems loaded against people of colour. The same issue exists in relation to gender, sexual identity, disability and so forth.

We may have beneficent intentions for assessing and making judgements in many areas. The same way that teachers are expected to assess children's ability for school streaming purposes, medics diagnose, and compile treatment protocols and Human Resources run recruitment drives. But we need to be cautious as it is only a short step to reducing people to just one aspect of their experience, and this is what the contributors explore in this part—one in relation to one's country of origin, a second in relation to race, a third in relation to sexual identity, and the fourth in relation to trans and non-binary allyship. While the reduction of people to groups *can* be helpful, contributors show that it is always complex and precarious, seldom completely good.

Parizad Bathai explores hate, a powerful emotion but one that, both individually and as members of a group, can be hard to deal with. We see people either getting caught up in it, or we shy away from our hate, ashamed to feel it, worried in case others would see us being hateful. It is a hard emotion to be subjected to, but Parizad offers us insight into the way hate is projected and experienced, especially when based on assumed cultural otherness.

Yetunde Ade-Serrano considers race, when and how one is made aware of race or the colour of one's skin and the meaning this may have individually and situationally. Yetunde reflects on the experience of being seen as different and the way this distances and separates people. Yetunde describes processes of engaging with, and humanising, the other, and the ways in which this is therapeutic—albeit oftentimes well outside of the formal structures of "therapy" as currently constructed. In this way, Yetunde engages with the questions Alison Greenwood raised in her earlier chapter about the status of rules and our responsibility to go beyond them.

Carter Jacobs offers an exploration of similar processes in relation to homo-negativity and in particular how this can manifest even within intimate relationships. He reminds us that it is not just heterosexuals who can be homophobic. We all grow up in a heterosexist society and as such are exposed to, and absorb, powerful, homo-negative attitudes. It is just that the LGBTQ person has to do the work to overcome (or at least manage) the structural and internalised discrimination. If not, it is toxic and LGBTQ people do the work of the aggressor for them.

The final chapter is by Julia Brewer who explores the complexity of allyship, and specifically Trans-allyship. By reflecting on her own experience in the most everyday of settings—on social media, in friendship groups and when being shown to a table in a restaurant—Julia notes both the prevalence of gendered assumptions and the tension that exist when trying to challenge these. How to challenge? When to? Might our involvement sometimes be clumsy or gauche and might allies sometimes "put their foot in it"? Her reflections lead, not to one correct way to be an ally, but to an exploration of the management of the tensions that arise in these efforts.

Drama of Phantom Hatred

Parizad Bathai

Scene 1

These days my hate is looking for new targets, as the old ones don't seem so hateful anymore. Over the years, the targets have changed. Some felt legitimate and righteous and some less so. Some of this hate turns inwards. The extras go to others. Sometimes, I feel justified to have hateful thoughts and sometimes I am ashamed. It seems I have no logical and reasonable control over this particular feeling. It is fresh, cold and brutal.

Gone are those days when our hatred was gloriously attached to the love for humanity and creation of a utopia. Imperialism and capitalism have triumphed and I am personally defeated.

In the first year of my MA studies at the department of English literature, we had an American lecturer. He was assigned to university as part of a programme called Fulbright by the USA.

P. Bathai (✉)
London, UK

Fulbright was an ideological set up to prevent university students becoming political. Arrogant and detached, as any home lecturer, he had extra flair to show his arrogance. He used to sit with his legs on the desk, never taught us literature but talked ideology. One day in his idiotic rambling, he said he used to teach in Pakistan and "They don't know how to laugh". I was so tempted to say "You get out of Pakistan and they will learn how to laugh." I quietly collected my books and walked towards the door. As I was leaving, he shouted "Hey! You don't like what I am saying? It is the truth", I didn't respond and left. At the end of the term I saw next to my name, the first failing mark of 0 (0 is F with more humiliation attached to it). I had never failed before or since in my academic studies.

I used to carry my resentment with some dignity. I took this big fat zero as an accolade for my fight against imperialism! Something to be proud of. I didn't approach anyone at the university to protest. No one dared to question him or check his marking and if they did, no one questioned a Fulbright agent from the USA. We didn't expect justice or fairness. But this was not the fault of Americans. This was the norm in our own country. For the 2nd year of the MA, he was still teaching the course. I decided not to continue. That summer, I came to the UK to stay with an English family. On the day of my departure at the airport, we saw each other. I never forget the triumphant smirk on his face.

I can't remember becoming hate-filled until I became political. At personal level, hate was not supposed to have a place in our internal world. We didn't dare express hate towards our parents or siblings. So, our hate looked around and searched in order to find a legitimate target. The standard route in our political life was, after declaring love for the dispossessed, was declaring hate for the imperialists. And I was personally wounded by one!

Like my lecturer, the foreign powers had full control over all aspects of our political lives. They trained dictators and torturers, organised coups, brought back kings who were trying to flee the popular uprising; they set up secret police and a brutal army.

These obvious acts of domination stopped us seeing if we were really capable of creating a democratic society. It blinded us to our own shortcomings.

Scene 2

These days my hatred has downgraded itself. Not being able to fight the bigger system, it wanders around and picks more manageable targets. I noticed that these days it tends to go after foreigners, foreigners like myself. "Why do they have to be so many of them? Why don't they learn to be more (English like me!?)" Why aren't they aware how foreign they are? Look what they have done to my reputation? It seems that I have worked very hard to be a good foreigner and enhance my image only to witness how it is sabotaged by other foreigners. "Why do they have to talk so loud?"

These thoughts don't last long but long enough for me to know that I blame other foreigners for becoming more aware, almost every day, that I am a foreigner. Their constant presence in the news has made it impossible for me to forget my fragile place in this world. Their presence is a constant reminder of how I am looked at. I hate my accent even more. A few years ago, I enrolled in a course for "accent softening" and all the tutor did was relaxation technique. Damn fool!

We don't like each other. "Can you please throw the rest out?" All foreigners in my street have voted for Brexit, all of them! Spanish, Portuguese, Italian, Irish, Polish and Romanians. I have heard them murmuring "too many of them, people have to go back!" We nod as we each have a particular group of people whom we like to hate. No one, and I mean the host country, points the finger of blame at us! No one suspects that foreigners could be so devious and hateful.

In my recent trip round the UK, Cathy the American tourist asked me where I was from. I know that in these circumstances, I have to add few words of comfort and apology after saying "I am from Iran **BUT** I live in the UK. I have lived in the UK for 40 years" I am trying to sooth any anxiety on their part. After my personal encounter with Mr Fulbright, I never saw another American for a long time. Then at my workplace and in my group tours I met individuals. Much to my surprise I really liked them. I could relate to them. Whoever I met I found likeable, warm, humorous, even left wing and innocent. I saw no malice in any of them. After 9/11, my hate emigrated to another group. I asked myself "do you want to live under imperialism or al-Qaida's regime?" The answer was clear cut.

After my reconciliation with the "Imperialists", you can imagine my shock when I saw a Fulbright smirk on Cathy's face. "Oh No!" I said to myself "You fool! Why did you say you were Iranian? You could have said Greek, or Italian or any old non- threatening nationality." I knew the damage was done. When I went back to the coach, I felt really hateful of myself and my stupidity, and I felt that old feeling which gives birth to hate: humiliation.

The matter became worse when she introduced me to her husband as he approached us "Honey, she is from Iran **BUT** she has been in the UK for a long time." It sounded to me "She is now germ free; she no longer has Ebola and she is no longer contagious." I had to remind myself that I started this. I wanted to reassure everyone that I am not a new arrival, that I have nothing to do with those people who trouble you. I didn't want to be hated. Considering that the majority in the tour were from the USA, I really wanted to be someone else. Being me felt wrong. Cathy's reassurance didn't comfort her husband so they both avoided me. In order to regain some dignity, I also ignored them and that felt better. To feel even better, I ignored the rest of them too.

Scene 3

The biggest portion of my resentment goes to my own country. Forty years after we blamed the west for not allowing us to have a democratic system, we are facing our own part in our failure. It is such a shame not to have anyone else to blame. Such a shame that our hate went around the globe and came back empty handed. Our impotent rage tries to find another hate figure. Our impotent rage cries out "Someone must put things right for us."

Scene 4

After a minor op under general anaesthetic, I opened my eyes and before I knew where I was and who I was I burst into tears. A Philippino nurse took my hand and asked "What's the matter dear?" I sobbed "I don't want to be a foreigner". She calmly responded "we all are."

I am stuck with my own kind!

Sometime ago, I read somewhere that in Poland where for many years after the war there were no Jews left, the anti-Semitic feelings were high. The writer compared this with a phenomenon of phantom pain when an amputee feels pain in limbs that are no longer there. Phantom hatred has no basis in reality. It just roams and lingers over someone or something for a while till the next scene.

The safest way for me to watch this drama is to send it to the orbit, watch it, understand it and acknowledge it but don't let it land. It can hover up there forever as a phantom of our marvellous mind.

Reflections from a Junkyard Room

Yetunde Ade-Serrano

Introduction

The idea that life today is dissimilar to what has happened in the past is foreign to me. I say this because the events we observe in our life now are a culmination of actions that have happened in the past. Yesterday's life can present differently today but everything that happened in the past has an impact on the present as it will in future, whether known or unknown.

While I do not have ready-made solutions to some of the questions I ponder, the aim is to highlight the experiences that have left me shackled to the past, the idea of vulnerability, my own power and the choices that enable or disable this.

I am not new to telling stories, but I have never told one like this before in this way. Although I am holding the space for my experiences, I am also aware that inadvertently I may be giving a voice to those who

Y. Ade-Serrano (✉)
London, UK

share similar experiences. Why does this have a bearing here? I do not want to minimise their experiences as I am not adequately equipped to fully represent them here because my voice is dominant. Even someone from a similar background to me who was born in my home country would have had a different experience growing up and would most likely have a different take on the assertions that I make. I acknowledge the power that I hold in my ability to tell a story using this platform, but my hope is that through this piece others can tell their own stories.

I plan to share thoughts and experiences from what I coin the junkyard room. This is conceived as thinking and experiences stored together often in a place in the mind and body. Within this storage system, I have images of various experiences preserved in bubbles. Some experiences are more significant than others and therefore a variation in the size of bubbles.

I think of the relevance of each experience and how much area the bubble takes up. Everyone has junk—even saying this prompts a memory. I remember going to a scrapyard for the very first time looking for a spare part for my car from cars that had mostly been involved in accidents. The severity of damage varied but I found some useful things that I was not looking for.

Growing Up and Beyond

Looking back on my childhood, I do not recollect having a concept of what it meant to be different because of my skin colour. I grew up relatively different to others in my immediate vicinity in so far as my mother's keenness on me having an education was concerned. In this respect, I grew up fortunate that this was possible. Those less well-off than us were treated differently, some even badly. The rationale for treating people differently or badly was not down to their skin colour. In the part of West Africa where I grew up, I was surrounded by different people. Within my family, we were a mix of multiple continents. The understanding of "race" I have today was not one I had as a child. Those with white skin were treated differently—they were revered. At the time, I thought this was because they travelled more than others in the family and therefore, they were special. Looking back, I did not have any appreciation for racial differences.

When families had problems or individuals within communities needed to resolve issues, the protocol was to sit with the elders of the family or community or speak to the priest. Doing this was an endeavour to iron out differences and come to a compromise that worked for everyone. People talked about the good, the bad and the ugly. The elders or priest gave direction, reminded people of the need to work together to achieve a common goal. It was not always cordial because there were times when individuals felt ostracised due to their unique beliefs, but people generally tended to come to an agreement. Outside of resolving issues, relationships were intimate, people knew each other particularly if you came from a small community. Our open-house policy meant friends and families could visit at any time, people ate together, drank together, danced and remained together in times of need.

Fast forward to today and living in London, I know the effect of having a different skin colour. The community spirit I perceived while growing up does not exist in London. It seems to me that every person roots for themselves. There are no visible elders in the community one can talk to. The church is present but not in the way I remember it. This may be because of the disconnection I feel—the priest and congregation do not engage in the same way I witnessed previously. I often wonder why?

Confronting Therapy

I met an old lady once on the train on my way back from a conference. We talked about her experiences in the academic world in the US, she told me about her children and about her life. I told her about mine and the conference I had just attended. We shared various experiences until we arrived at the last stop. The exchange on the train was so engaging we carried on, sitting in a coffee shop until many hours had passed. We swapped numbers and email and promised to keep in touch. I found this experience therapeutic—not because I had something to resolve psychologically. It was rather an emotional and spiritual connection. On my part, I was not inhibited, I felt no shame, I was free to be myself and I immediately trusted her. I think it was the same for her. We had met in an authentic place and all of the bubbles in the junkyard room were relevant. Simplistically, this was therapy. Reflecting on the memories of growing up, it strikes me that the elders and the priests were engaging in "therapy" with the community.

From a practice point of view, therapy today is perceived differently. Therapy is seen as a process of resolving psychological issues, you (individuals, couples or groups) sit in a room in front a therapist who will help you fix the problem. There is a set day, time and room in which it occurs—it is prescriptive. The rigidity of this structure is probably about the ramifications of not practicing safely. At the same time, "the encounter" does not have to be practiced this way for it to be called therapy. Thinking about what I know of therapy and my experience with the lady on the train, several things occurred—openness, disclosure, empathy, curiosity and positive regard. Encountering her was intimate and real. Is this not synonymous with the encountering in a therapy room? If it is, does the interaction contravene the safety of the therapy room as we define it today? Were ethical codes broken in so relating? What about the cradle of confidentiality given that our conversation was on a train journey with others within hearing distance?

Are we missing the relevance of everyday therapeutic engaging?

Therapy is the junction at which the old way of talking meets the new, it is the replication of the old within a fundamentally similar world. People have the same issues, sometimes they utilise the relationships with elders or priests or seek to sit with a therapist. One of my favourite authors says, "effective therapy consists of alternating sequence: evocation and experiencing of affect followed by analysis and integration of affect[1]". Therapy is the ability to connect, perhaps reflect, experience the other person in their entirety during the experience. We may analyse the experience during or after it has happened. Indeed, this speaks to the basis of human connection—whatever relationship in which the encountering occurs.

---

[1] Yalom (2002, p. 72).

This is how I see therapy, the privilege of re-enabling the human connection, creating the space and providing the ingredients needed to facilitate openness, intimacy, regard, empathy etc.

Blackness and Therapy

Regardless of arguments around "Blackness" or "Race" as social constructs, the reality is, society distinguishes between White and non-White people by ascribing non-White in most cases as Black. Of course, there are variations of Black. I don't know anything other than what I am and so I am proud to be Black, my skin colour isn't black at all but a mixture of hazel and milk chocolate. I choose to describe myself as a child of the world because of the multiple facets of who I am which is not confined within anyone culture or locality. I am aware of my privilege, it does not define who I am but facilitates interactions with different people. "We learn best about ourselves and our behaviours through personal participation in interaction combined with observation and analysis of that interaction[2]".

One of the times I experienced racism, an old white lady told me to "go back to where you came from". Reflecting now on that memory, I am not confused as to what occurred nor am I surprised, but I am always shocked when it happens—barefaced racism. At that time, this old white lady lived in the flat underneath me with her grown up son. She came to the door one day with a complaint about something she alleged I had done. I tried to explain I had no idea what she was talking about, but she was too angry to listen, hurling abuse at me. My initial thought was if I pushed this fragile frame down the stairs, I could kill her and consequently, I would be arrested. Multiple questions went through my mind—would she have told a White person to go back to where they came from? Was I being overly sensitive? Was she being racist or just angry? Why was her anger directed at me when others lived in the building? This experience was one too many where my skin colour was referenced within a conflict situation. I was left feeling that being Black

---

[2] Yalom (2002, p. 65).

was an issue. In conversation with others, who identify as Black the narrative is similar. The experiences reinforce the idea that in London, you are treated differently because of your skin colour.

Blatant racism exists, although there are shifts in its manifestation. In my professional world, I give lectures on covert and overt racism. I talk with people about the implicit racist expressions termed "microaggression". I wonder though, is this just a softening of the blows dealt by such behaviours? Unconcealed racism has not gone away, and I feel angry at the thought that some think it has disappeared. Microaggression in whatever form is subtle—that is the defining characteristic—but the impact on the person receiving it is far from understated.

Another experience I had was during my "A" levels. I was studying 3 sciences, wanting to fulfil a childhood dream of being a medical doctor, I was told by my personal tutor who had to sign my application form that "people like you should be catering assistants and not gynaecologists". This person so happened to be a White middle-aged man. This was an extremely traumatic and life-changing event. On reflection, at the time, while devastating, I did not perceive it as anything other than the truth. Hence, what I learnt was that because of my skin colour, I am less than; I do not, therefore, have access to the resources I require to be what or who I want to be. These experiences are part of my history and links with my ancestor's history—my great grandparent was sold into slavery. In my thinking, these two events are aligned. I carry with me all these experiences whether direct (they happened to me) or indirect (others that I am a part of).

Thinking of the conscious and unconscious ways I process my skin colour as an issue, I wonder who has the issue? Me? Or others? I have sophisticated ways of thinking and analysing my behaviour in relation to others, although of course, "splitting" can occur. At the same time, it is quite a difficult task when I have objective evidence to substantiate the experiences I have. And this is the tricky side of being on the receiving end of racism—I constantly question whether it is real or whether the problem is located within my consciousness. A potential outcome of gaslighting, especially when contextualised within power dynamics. This can trigger a sense of not being good enough among other inadequacies.

In cases like this, the hesitancy to sit in front of a therapist is about a lack of trust. Will a White therapist treat me like I am less than? Will they find within my damaged self a salvageable me like I did when looking in the scrapyard for car parts? Will they understand where I am coming from? Will they react defensively? Will I need to defend myself in a place where I am meant to feel safe? Even when the therapist is from a Black background, sometimes these questions can come to mind. The Black therapist is often also dealing with their own internalised racism. For these reasons, often people who look like me choose not to seek therapeutic help.

On the other hand, it is sometimes important to have a frank conversation, even if they illuminate divisions. I recently attended a one-day conference where speakers talked about the experience of racism and the power dynamics within those experiences. The speakers were all different in the way that they looked—some were White, and others were from Black and Asian communities—like the attendees. One of the speakers, a White man, in his mid to late fifties I would guess, recounted an experience where he and his colleagues from Black and Asian communities were conducting research in a nameless country. He stated that participants of the research refused to engage his colleagues because they thought that he—the White man—oversaw the research. This is a common experience where Black people tend to be seen as followers rather than leaders. Within this conference space, where we were learning about racism and having open conversations, there was still an air of defensiveness. The White people in the room found it difficult to understand how the Black and Asian people in the room felt. We ended up in a divided situation.

The Dominance of the English Language

When I began telling this story, there were probably words or sentences that resonated with you. Some may have repelled you. The fact is, the same word can mean multiple things to one person let alone multiple people. What does it mean when someone says, "people like you should be catering assistants?" Does it mean women? Young person?

Black person? Or a combination of? How mindful are we when we use language like this—be it spoken or unspoken? Is there a conscious acknowledgement of how language can shape and continue to structure discrimination? Perhaps we just don't think about it.

I too get caught out in my thought processes in so far as being aware of how language often moulds how I think and make decisions. One of my trigger words is "monkey". As an animal, their shape, their pose, so beautiful and gracious. What can I say—beauty is in the eye of the beholder. However, as a word, the association exists in how it is used as a derogatory term for Black people. There are many examples—see complaints in football alone. An article in the Guardian purported that there was a 50% rise in football-related racist incidents which included referring to Black players as monkeys or making monkey noises at them.[3] One that I remember been in the news was the racist remarks against Raheem Sterling, who played for Manchester City at the time when he scored against Bournemouth in 2018. Two Manchester City fans used racist language against him. In another example, Antonio Rudiger who currently plays for Chelsea was subjected to monkey chants from Tottenham Hotspur fans in late 2019. There is no justification for using language in this way, obviously!

A while ago, I read an article published in 1973, nearly 50 years ago—Burgest said

> "language as a potent force of our society goes beyond being merely a communicative device. Language not only expresses ideas and concepts but may actually shape them. Often the process is completely *unconscious with the individual concerned unaware of the influence of the spoken or written expression upon his thought process.*[4] "

See what I mean about the old overlaying the new? This written nearly 50 years ago is very appropriate today!

The dominance of the English language is noted in Burgest's emphasis on how language can shape ideas and concepts. In the English language,

---

[3] Bassam (2020).
[4] Burgest (1973, p. 37). Italics added for emphasis.

there is a vast contrast in how black and white is perceived. Black is synonymous to "bad" while "White" is good. In the media, for example, headlines often depict White perpetrators utilising soft narratives compared to hard hitting stereotypical headlines that portray a negative impression of Black perpetrators. In addition, the domination of the English language is connected to colonialism and the number of territories that were inhabited by English speaking empires.

We use language to communicate, and it is extremely useful in expressing what we feel or think or in trying to make sense of the world. At the same time, language, particularly English as a dominant discourse, is used to alienate Black communities often by those in positions of greater power and influence. Do you remember when Donald Trump tweeted about Black and Asian congresswomen representatives? He claimed they should "go back to where they came from". Was this because he felt threatened? Or he just wanted to ridicule them? Or was he recounting the use of language that he had been indoctrinated to? Just like when the old White lady told me to go back to where I came from.

This kind of language belittles a person, it penetrates so deep, the length and breadth of it too painful. It triggers experiences that have passed from one generation to another—not purposefully taught, like you would teach the alphabets to a toddler—but unconsciously assumed. I know the words that quashed my dreams, my hopes and my aspirations. Christina Aguilera's[5] song "Beautiful" says "… words can't bring me down". The truth is, words demolished the house I once built. The pain is not mine alone, as words used against others like me is forever a sore spot. Like bell hooks once said "… like desire, language disrupts, refuses to be contained within boundaries. It speaks itself against our will, in words and thoughts that intrude, even violate the most private spaces of mind and body[6]".

---

[5] Aguilera (2002).
[6] Hooks (1994, p. 167).

The Shackles of Vulnerability

I want to briefly talk to how history has played out. As I mentioned before, my ancestors were sold into slavery. I was not physically present at the time. However, I do carry the burden of historic trauma they experienced which would have ranged from lack of material wealth, captivity, gendered suppression to physical and psychological oppression. This list is by no means exhaustive. In my experiences today, while not the same circumstances, these historical oppressions still exist and I suffer the same consequences—loss of my identity, loss of my voice, not belonging, reduced access to resources, feelings of inferiority, feeling that I am constantly under a microscope, the examples are endless. Does history play with human evolution by repeating itself? How do I unconsciously contribute to the legacy of this history?

Growing up, I have no memory of been told about my ancestors or their history. I found out about the history of my name and its origins by accident. A dinner lady at my secondary school prompted my investigations. Can you imagine what it feels like to be told of your lineage by a stranger? Knowing what I know about the history of my ancestors albeit not in the detail I would like has left "something" within me. On one hand, I am delighted that a stranger recognised me in my name. This tells me my ancestors were well known and regarded and left a legacy behind. On the other hand, I have this sense of nothingness. I didn't know them and there is not enough acknowledgement about them and the great work that they did—the information has been buried in archives. This shackle of vulnerability is present in my engagement with my family, friends and colleagues. This history plus my personal experiences reinforce what was then, what is now and what is to come.

How do we break free from these shackles? This is a recurrent question I ask myself. I am loath to suggest that forgetting my history is an option because it isn't. Is it about forgiving my history? I contend it is not about letting go of the pain or giving a pass to how we have constructed the narratives around those that perpetuate the problems. Perhaps it is about learning what our weaknesses and strengths are and trusting in them in so far as recognising the power and privilege this gives us. The power that I have exists within the choices that I make, good, bad or indifferent.

Furthermore, the freedom to execute this power I think is the key to breaking these shackles.

Remember my journey on the train and the connection with the stranger? She was a White old lady. I have had my fair share of not so great experiences with White old ladies. I stored these experiences in their bubbles in my junkyard. These experiences would have been activated given the profile of this woman. But they did not. As you read this, you will have your own thoughts and analyses as to why these experiences were not brought to the fore with this woman on the train. I do not want to contribute to that. What I will say is, this experience on the train dilutes all my negative experiences with old White ladies. There is a possibility I can continue to find useful nuggets of connections within the junkyard like I did when I was looking for the spare parts so many years ago.

I often listen to Brené Brown's[7] Ted talk. I get what she means about vulnerability. She titles her talk "the power of vulnerability" which underpins shame and fear, preventing connection from occurring between people. While I am moved by most of her assertions, I also now name vulnerability "a shackle". It is a historical bondage that I continually try to break free from. I am not scared to walk towards vulnerability because it has already captured me.

I want to acknowledge the privileges I have attained since my journey to becoming me started, a lot of people have contributed to my learning. I always have the power to decide, but fear and priority given to the needs of others sometimes hinder my use of it—the fear that I was not good enough, the fear that I was not well versed enough, the fear of failing. I realised some time back that I could use my voice, despite the fears, and that the development for me and others in so doing, outweighed any negative consequences that could emerge.

In my junkyard room, there are many bubbles of varying sizes. I often fumble around looking for appropriate experiences to base my decisions on. Those who engage with me a little or extensively share in the experiences that I bring. I continue in my journey constantly discovering the multitudes of myself regardless of what is visible to the eyes of others.

---

[7] Brown (2010).

I have multiple bubbles as you know, sometimes they bounce up and become triggered memories. Other times they do not. My privilege is being ok with the choices I make; I sit on top of the world as I burst the bubbles of memories I no longer require and which take up space. All that encompasses who I am is ok. I enjoy the privilege of having a multi-ethnic DNA, an understanding that is different from others but also sharing commonalities. It is a privilege to share my voice and sometimes I am heard.

The junkyard room, have you found yours? What can you discover?

Acknowledgements With God, all things are possible.

To my ancestors who continue to pave my way.

To the men in my life, the one who grounds me and the one who is the yin to my yang.

References

Aguilera, C. (2002). *Beautiful*. https://www.youtube.com/watch?v=eAfyFTzZDMM.
Bassam, T. (2020, January 30). Sharp rise in football racism as incident go up by more than 50% in one year. *The Guardian*. https://www.theguardian.com/football/2020/jan/30/football-related-racist-incidents-sharp-rise-police-kick-it-out. Downloaded on 22 January 20.
Brown, B. (2010, June). *The power of vulnerability* [Video]. Ted Talk. https://www.ted.com/talks/brene_brown_the_power_of_vulnerability?language=en#t-1200341. Downloaded on 22 January 21.
Burgest, D. R. (1973). The racist use of English language. *The Black Scholar, Black Media, 5*(1), 37–45.
Hooks, b. (1994). *Teaching to transgress: Education as the practice of freedom*. Routledge.
Yalom, I. D. (2002). *The gift of therapy*. HarperCollins.

"I'm Not as Bad as You"

Carter Jacobs

We were jerking each other off, something we did on a regular basis, when I leant in to kiss him.

'No' he said, 'Uh, Uh. I'm not as bad as you'.

No beat was skipped, we continued pumping away enthusiastically, becoming more and more excited until we each reached a climax. That was cool apparently. What wasn't cool was feeling something for each other, showing tenderness or affection.

We were teenagers, hard-ons more common than blinking, desire more urgent than pride. Maybe that's why that moment didn't stop us finishing each other off. But as we cleaned up, that statement seared itself into my psyche. Its impact has faded but not completely. It is still there, evident if you know where to look. In that one statement, Dylan

---

C. Jacobs (✉)
London, UK

had given voice to a lifetime of brainwashing, the 16 years we'd already endured, and the decades more that were to come.

Tired from our exertions, we didn't think about any of this, our encounters were just something that "happened". A lot. As long as it wasn't talked about, or even thought about in any depth, it was fine. We would revert to conversation about how the Yankees were doing, our homework or who (which girl) we might ask to the summer formal.

Pay that moment any attention, the attention I *wanted* us to give it, and there lay the route to ridicule, isolation and potentially violence. Thinking about it, or even riskier, *talking* about it, would make it real. I yearned for that, yet how could I? Everyone knew that if you *flaunted* it punishment was all but guaranteed. You knew what would follow; "Faggot!" "Queer!" And we didn't need to *hear* that every day, it was *felt* all the time. Hate was just off stage, waiting in the wings, ready to be called forth should you transgress.

I worried. We heard about hate and violence all the time—James Zapporloti—Dead. Paul Broussard—Dead. Allan Schindler—Dead. Brandon Teena—Dead. I hadn't been assaulted, not physically, but threat was everywhere, so palpable that I would worry myself to sleep. What if people found out? The absence of overt violence—so far—didn't fix anything. It was better than if the jocks had come my way, gay bashing for fun, but when hatred goes underground it doesn't mean it has gone, or it has no effect. No, its effect is insidious.

Nowadays people know you're not *allowed* to beat the crap out of someone because of their sexuality; there are sanctions strong enough to make *most* people think twice. But it's no guarantee.

March 2014—the rapper Jipsta was attacked with his partner on the New York City subway
June 2016—The Pulse Nightclub massacre. 49 people were killed and more than 50 injured.
August 2019—a man in the Bronx was attacked with a hammer and thrown on to subway tracks as the assailant yelled "faggot[1]".

---

[1] Denny (2019).

And it's not only in the US of course.

Anti-gay hate crime rose after the UK's 2016 Brexit referendum.[2] Uganda has ongoing legislative attempts to outlaw same sex sexuality.[3] And there's the Chechnya purge. And Erdogoan and Bolsanaro too.

Dylan and I didn't have to experience a hate crime, be beaten or suspended from school to feel threatened, the simplest of slights were a reminder of the risks of being different. While it was tantalising to see Prince and other rock stars flout the rules and make androgyny fashionable, on the street an active, physical masculinity, untainted by any hint of femininity remained a requirement; the rejection of subtlety, fragility or emotion the norm.

The misogynistic foundations of homophobia are woven into the fabric of our lives but help no-one—it diminishes women's worth, cleaves men's emotional depth from them and poisons the environment for us all. It underpins the out-of-control violence directed at our trans and non-binary siblings too.

The more subtle forms of attack are even less effectively policed; in fact, it seems that we reward those who hate—the class clown belittles the queer kid to get his laughs; Governor Pence was elected Vice President after presiding over cuts to HIV funding and a rise in infection[4]; the UK Prime Minister wins by a landslide despite using homophobic (and sexist and racist) language[5]; and Brazil's Jair Bolsanaro rails against "gay tourism[6]". The list goes on, impacting our emotional, social and cultural wellbeing.

The everyday slights and woundings are very prevalent. Yet if you call them out, there are claims of "cancel culture", that the bully had no "conscious" intent to hurt, they're "just" locker-room talk, politician's

---

[2] Antjoule (2016).
[3] OutRight Action International (n.d.).
[4] Kalichman (2017).
[5] Bienkov (2019).
[6] Phillips and Kaiser (2019).

"colourful language[7]" or closer to home the rejection of my kiss and that comment, "I'm not as bad as you".

Complain and people ask, "So what's the big deal?" "It's no different to what anyone has to go through" they say. They gaslight you, turn it on its head. They reframe bullying as benevolence, "it prepares them for the real world" they say. Teasing geeky boys is meant to "make a man out of them"? And it supposedly prepares girls for a lifetime of their bodies being scrutinised—it's "natural" apparently. The argument seems to be, it happens to everyone so get over it, "teasing" is a part of life, never did "us" any harm. "Man up and deal with it".

But No. The ubiquity of these dehumanising slights does not make it right. Habituate people to aggression early so as to limit trauma of later violence? Nonsense, it's not a vaccine. Aggression does the opposite, it primes us for what is to come, wounds us early and keeps an unnecessary level of stress.

If it wasn't so damaging the persistence of this negativity might be fascinating; What is this preoccupation about? Why does it happen? What maintains it? More positively, who *gains* from it? How can we make more use of the alliances that exist between all of us who face these attacks. Racism, transphobia, misogyny and other forms of discriminatory microaggressions *share* an enormous amount too.

Whether the threat is overt or covert, to avoid the full impact of hate, like other minorities, LGBTQ folk become attuned to it, mindful of it, familiar with its various shapes, forms and tones. It is never a singular, or static, experience. Not only did I, and so many of my contemporaries, have to watch out for signs of rejection or aggression from others, we started to do it to ourselves. Slavish adherence to hypermasculine bodies, forever critical, always feeling the need to change—tighten this, loosen that, tone the pecs. Internalised hate morphs into interpersonal attacks as we sometimes see in queer communities when we belittle our camp brothers and butch sisters. Thank god for RuPaul and all of the courageous Queens on whose shoulders she stands.

So yes, those who are demonised and aggressed against learn the quixotic nature of scrutiny and the fact that judgement never goes

---

[7] Merrick (2019).

away—it's always there, so we study it, and absorb it. It helps us survive. But the need to be alert, avoid and manage it means you become preoccupied with it, and then anxiety follows. Not only is that painful, what Robert Hopcke[8] refers to as soul murder, but there's a double-whammy. That protective vigilance is pathologised, turned against us so we're perceived as paranoid or as "grievance collectors[9]". It's a magnificent sleight of hand, the recipient of the prejudice becomes the problem, not the perpetrator—"You can't take a joke" they say, "I didn't mean it" they moan, "You're making something out of nothing" they accuse.

Structural issues matter as they normalise perceptions and practices that should not be normalised. It's there in politics—Reagan's refusal to speak of AIDS essentially hamstrung research and treatment, allowing the epidemic to claim so many lives, and the 2017 erasing of LGBTQ information from the White House website allowed the needs of queer people to be overlooked—again. Poland's "Gay Free Zones" are a threat too.

This matters.

In the leafy, progressive suburbs of Westchester, Dylan and I did our best, each of us trying to find ways out of this web. For a while, my way was to watch and emulate, rock stars, movie icons and the popular guys around me. I remember cycling home from the movies. It was summer and I was imagining myself as Brad Pitt, wielding my hairdryer as he did in *Thelma and Louise*, and all the while being effortlessly attractive to, and attracted by, women. That would be normal, I thought. "Normal", such a desirable, all pervasive yet ultimately meaningless concept. But yeh, I wanted to be Brad, that would be so much more preferable than having to learn to be comfortable in my own skin, a skin that would attract shock and hate should people know of its desires in my small town, small in size and small in mind.

I tried to identify with the boys who seemed at ease with girls—one day I would emulate Jimmy, the tough kid from our neighbourhood, another I'd want to be Billy, smart and bright, and often I would try to be like Logan.

---

[8] Hopcke (2002).
[9] Socarides (1995).

Oh Logan! Logan was calm, quiet with a great sense of humour. Everyone liked him and he moved from crew to crew effortlessly. He became my template to being straight, or at least to passing. It didn't hurt that he had great hair and cute eyes either. Oh! And a chest that gave me the shivers … it was at that point that I realised that this strategy wasn't fool proof. Nor was it healthy, trying to be like someone else. I didn't realise it at the time but activities like this are more than just some adolescent "trying on" of identities, they were a rejection of my essence, damaging my self-esteem, affecting my choice of partners and, for the longest time, my availability for love and intimacy.

Picking at the Scar

Today I am healthy and not particularly closeted. I'm out to my family, friends and at work. Being white, male and bright I live a life of significant privilege, yet still I carry that scar, sometimes thinking that I wasn't as good as someone else, simply because of who I was attracted to.

Even though I have challenged the attacks on us, protested and been active, it's not a one shot deal. I was outraged about the Defence of Marriage Act (DOMA) and argued against it in debate-soc, albeit I focussed on *civil* rights rather than *gay* rights. In Grad School, I was vocal about Lawrence vs Texas[10] but couldn't shake the worry about being seen as too political. I heard about Section 28 on the other side of the pond, an abhorrent policy that made it illegal for teachers to "promote" homosexuality, a forerunner of Russia's 2013 law—but about that I was simply relieved that I wasn't going to be a teacher in the UK.

Why was I quiet? I sometimes wonder. Too tired maybe? Being a representative is exhausting. Felt it wasn't my argument? Or did I absorb political spin as fact, not even seeing how far and wide the toxicity of the times spreads. Or was it a manifestation of the shame I was so well trained to feel?

---

[10] Texas had tried to say sex in private was not a right for LGBT people. It was struck down by this case.

My scar started to hurt recently. We were at a wedding, in a beautiful cliff-top hotel, overlooking the pacific. I knew most of the guests, a progressive left-leaning lot—probably Hillary voters back in the day, maybe even some for Bernie. I could let my guard down for a while.

As we sat outside, enjoying the warm summer evening, some locals were drawn to us, possibly by the idea of tipsy fresh-faced out-of-towners, looking for love—or at least, feeling a little horny. Two guys started to hit on several of the women, and soon the nature of the wedding was mentioned, there being two brides. "No shit" was the response of one, followed by "Oh, so not a real wedding then" from the other. That stung. I haven't seen Dylan since our college days, but it was like he had just spoken again. This time it was public. This time it was confronted. It was no longer two 16 year olds struggling with the closet.

I didn't need to say anything though, as several others called bullshit first. "Dude, I didn't mean nothing by it" was the response to one woman, our annoyance viewed as an "over-reaction". No evidence that these guys recognised their thoughtlessness, or the fact that they were doing violence to the spirit of the occasion. Thankfully the wedding couple were oblivious elsewhere, but still. Not cool.

More sadly though, despite the resistance, it lingered. It wasn't Dylan's return, or even really those two locals, it was me picking at the scar—I did it the other day as I was taking my morning cocktail too. I caught myself wistfully pondering if I would've been spared my HIV infection had I been straight?

The Dylans of the world, the opportunistic locals move on, but this is what the stigmatised are left with, the need to consistently be aware, to make the effort to catch the self-critical thoughts, to challenge the view that tells you your normal isn't normal, or that your delight is disgusting. It isn't. And I know that. But the impact of homophobia is deep rooted and has it's effect, the warding off of which is often a life-long project. Thankfully these moments of feeling worse than others are more limited and increasingly infrequent.

Life has gotten so much better.

It Does Get Better

As I write this in 2021, it's clear that there is more to do, especially with the regressive legislation we have seen these last four years killing off LGBT protections one by one.[11] But things can, and do, get better and when they do it is just, and it is wonderful. While there is concern about the newly reconstituted Supreme Court, we mustn't forget that Romer v Evans was beat down. Equal marriage was confirmed across the country. Similarly, the same UK parliament that put Section 28 into legislation, eventually overturned that poisonous education policy (in 2003). They also agreed equal marriage in most parts of the UK in 2013, enacted it in 2014 and made it nationwide in 2019 when it became law in Northern Ireland. We have LGBT representation in Hollywood and on TV, both as bit parts and as main characters and people still tune in, the world hasn't turned to brimstone and fire. While there is still much to do across the continent, teens and young people are confidently being themselves in greater and greater numbers and thriving as they do.

I smile, as I remember the delight I experienced when, in the midst of passion, I risked leaning in again only to have my partner respond, meeting my lips with his. Tongues tasting, thrusting themselves into each others' mouths. Instead of rejection, there was a shared desire, a communing. Joy—and justice—in these moments of unguarded intimacy, where desire is known and reciprocal, and affection and even love are not only allowed but are met, wanted and celebrated.

References

Antjoule, N. (2016). *The hate crime report 2016: Homophobia, biphobia and transphobia in the UK*. Galop.

Bienkov, A. (2019, November 22). Boris Johnson called gay men 'tank-topped bumboys' and black people 'piccaninnies' with 'watermelon smiles'. *Business Insider*. https://www.businessinsider.com/boris-johnson-record-sexist-hom

---

[11] The National Center for Transgender Equality, (n.d.) and Cook (2020).

ophobic-and-racist-comments-bumboys-piccaninnies-2019-6?r=US&IR=T. Downloaded on 8 January 2020.

Cook, C. (2020, June 30). *Trump signs anti-LGBTQ child welfare executive order*. Lambda Legal. https://www.lambdalegal.org/blog/20200630_trump-admin-child-welfare-executive-order. Downloaded 12 November 2020.

Denny, A. (2019, August 28). Brooklyn man charged with hate crime for homophobic stabbing attack, *New York Post*. https://nypost.com/2019/08/28/brooklyn-man-charged-with-hate-crime-for-homophobic-stabbing-attack/. Downloaded on 8 January 2020.

Hopcke, R. H. (2002). *Jung, Jungians and homosexuality*. Resource Publications.

Kalichman, S. C. (2017). Pence, Putin, Mbeki and their HIV/AIDS-Related crimes against humanity: Call for social justice and behavioral science advocacy *AIDS and Behavior, 21*, 963–967. https://doi.org/10.1007/s10461-017-1695-8 https://link.springer.com/content/pdf/10.1007/s10461-017-1695-8.pdf. Downloaded on 8 January 2020.

Merrick, R. (2019, November 28). Tory minister defends Boris Johnson's use of 'bum boys' term. *The Independent*. https://www.independent.co.uk/news/uk/politics/boris-johnson-bum-boys-homophobic-free-speech-election-tory-lgbt-a9224491.html. Downloaded 18 December 2019.

OutRight Action International. (2019, October 10). Uganda threatens to re-introduce "Anti-Homosexuality Act". https://outrightinternational.org/content/uganda-plans-re-introduce-anti-homosexuality-act. Downloaded 8 January 2020.

Phillips, T. & Kaiser, A. J. (2019, April 26). Brazil must not become a 'gay tourism paradise', says Bolsonaro. *The Guardian*. https://www.theguardian.com/world/2019/apr/26/bolsonaro-accused-of-inciting-hatred-with-gay-paradise-comment. Downloaded 18 December 2019.

Socarides, C. W. (1995). *Homosexuality: A freedom too far*. Adam Margrave Books.

The National Center for Transgender Equality. (n.d). *The discrimination administration*, https://transequality.org/the-discrimination-administration. Downloaded on 22 January 2021.

Is There Something You Need to Tell Us?

Julia Brewer

"Is there something you need to tell us? ;-)"

This comment, beneath my Facebook post about transgender rights, made me angry. What were they trying to say? That if I was posting about an issue, it must affect me personally? That if I *was* transgender, there was a "need" to "admit" to it, like a shameful secret? The winking face emoji really annoyed me too. It was teasing apparently, but I felt there was an allusion to some kind of assumed in-joke between assumed cisgender[1] people, that being anything but cis would be something to be

---

[1] 'Cisgender' refers to people who identify with the gender they were assigned at birth. The diversity of identities beyond cisgender cannot neatly be reduced to a single term. Doing so is problematic as it can render the experiences of those who do not identify with it invisible. "Trans and non-binary" serves as an imperfect umbrella term to describe people who do not identify with the gender they were assigned at birth, including those who identify outside the binary categories "male" and "female".

J. Brewer (✉)
Coventry, UK

mocked for. A window opened into the kinds of pointed and discriminative interactions trans and non-binary people regularly navigate and the anger I felt at this injustice was loud and obvious. I stewed on the comment for some time. The more I did, the more I noticed something sticky in how I was feeling, there was something beyond the anger, something hiding behind it. I felt nervous, vulnerable somehow, and I soon realised what was in the stickiness—I didn't want people to think I was trans or non-binary myself.

A wave of shame came over me. The assumptions within the Facebook comment that I was outraged by appeared to be residing in some form within me too. I was alarmed by my discovery and having uncovered it I felt an urge to deny it. To re-bury it. How could I simultaneously feel so strongly about championing trans and non-binary rights and fighting prejudice, while holding some of that prejudice myself? What had I internalised and how might it be playing out elsewhere? I knew that some form of internalised transphobia[2] was a common experience among the trans and non-binary people I knew, but I had somehow developed an assumption that this internalisation was something that didn't—or couldn't—apply to me. That as a self-identified ally of the trans and non-binary community, and someone committed to rejecting such gender norms, I had somehow escaped the reality of being embedded in a cultural context, which inevitably leaves its marks on a deep unconscious level. The marks I had recognised here were uncomfortable to look at, but they could only be transformed if I attended to them. And so, a sharpened focus came. An opening up to the marks, scars and bruises, wherever they hid, as unconscious bias, prejudice and fear. I needed to do this to bring them into the light where I could examine them properly.

The volume of that immediate, familiar anger initially drowned out the quieter, less familiar parts of my response. Of course, it did. It's easy to make noise about things I don't agree with, the experiences I feel angry about. It's much harder to look inwardly and make noise about what I find there. So, what was within me? What was in that flash of fear that

---

[2] A discomfort with one's own gender non-conforming identity brought about by internalising society's rigid gender norms and expectations.

arose with the thought that someone might be questioning my gender identity?

"Is there something you need to tell us?"

Yes, I think there is.

I had been posting about trans and non-binary issues fairly regularly and having more conversations with friends and acquaintances about working in the field of gender diversity. It struck me that my own gender identity might be a common question in people's minds and this thought brought a sense of a spotlight being cast on me. Standing in its startling beam I felt on show, aware of a gaze I did not recognise. I felt highlighted as someone or something different and I feared the potential ostracisation that might come in being Othered. I felt a deep knot in my stomach, a heavy tension in my chest. In that moment, I felt isolated, out in the cold, as though a blanket that had been providing me with warmth and comfort had been suddenly whisked away leaving me exposed and vulnerable. But, that cold, tense, isolating fear was momentary, the discrimination only imagined. I was able to pull that blanket of cisgender privilege back over myself and not have to face the reality of such discrimination and abuse. The feeling, although transient, was helpfully quite powerful. I had previously understood myself to be inherently privileged, as someone for whom the gender I was assigned at birth, and cultural rules and assumptions around it, more or less work. I was confronted by the extent to which I take this for granted. Scrutiny had woken me up from a deep, comfortable slumber. As I now sat, awake and tuned in to the sensation of this blanket, I considered how enduring, exhausting and harmful exposure might be without this protective layer to retreat beneath.

"Is there something you need to tell us?"

Yes. And it's something about privilege.

A real awkwardness arose in me when acknowledging the extent of my privilege. An awkwardness I have grappled with in trying to make sense of what it means to be an ally. Who even am I to engage with and speak on matters I have no experience of? What place does a cisgender, heteronormative, person have here? This awkwardness was not new to me, but I was meeting it from a different perspective, with greater awareness of the significant layers of privilege I hold. It struck me that as someone who ultimately benefits from a culture that oppresses others, I have a fundamental responsibility to engage. A responsibility to be a part of highlighting and dismantling discriminatory systems, both within and beyond myself.

With the gathering momentum of the Black Lives Matter movement in recent years, it is being more widely recognised as not good enough for white people to identify themselves "not racist" and label themselves as outside the problems of racism. I see more conversations opening up about racism not being an issue just for people of colour to grapple with, but for all of us to engage with, in a self-reflective way. It seems there is some catching up for us to do in terms of transphobia. Having said this, I don't think it's helpful to position these as separate conversations. The reality is that the more forms of marginalisation a person faces, the more danger they face. To understand this, we just have to look at the experiences of transfeminine people of colour. Intersecting experiences of racism, sexism, homophobia, biphobia, transphobia and transmisogyny give rise to horrifying and disproportionate levels of violence. Fatal violence. So, yes, there has been an awkwardness to grapple with at times in my journey as an ally, but the responsibility is clear, not to shy away from, but to actively engage in conversations that are literally a matter of life and death.

So, it is not a question of *whether* we are positioned to engage with trans and non-binary issues, but *how*. Despite having connected to a strong sense of responsibility, I am learning that understanding the "how" here is complicated. I want to be the best ally I can be, but a part of me can feel like an imposter. It's not that the imposter feeling is misplaced or unhelpful. It keeps me alert and reflective with regard to the limitations or even potential for harm my positioning brings. It reminds me for example of the possibility, even with the best of intentions, of replicating colonial dynamics that have historically existed between marginalised and dominant groups. The privileged, with no lived experience of such marginalisation, apparently somehow "know better" and use this "knowing better" to liberate the oppressed. The grandiosity! This is not liberation, and if this is the historic experience of marginalised groups, I have to be sensitive to the possibility of my engagement being experienced in this way.

No one can possibly know better about the experiences, challenges, strengths and needs of trans and non-binary people than those people themselves. With this in mind, I have tried to look to the voices of trans and non-binary people as my compass throughout my journey as an ally. If I'm focusing on these voices, I am less at risk of imposing my own meaning onto other people's experiences. Although it is crucial that these voices remain my starting point and central focus, I have come to recognise that holding any position too rigidly can be unhelpful. For a long time, I was so desperate not to replicate any harmful dynamics or impose my frame of reference, that I denied my own experience altogether. On some level, I believed if I didn't share experience with a minority group, my experience didn't matter. What this extreme position crucially misses is that my experience is my only way of engaging with the world. If I shut it off, I shut off my ability to identify marks and scars. I block my route to reflection and learning and ultimately my ability to develop as an ally. If I turn towards my experience, I find a route into deeper connection with those who have experiences that might be very different to mine.

After the Facebook comment and the self-examination that followed, I began to notice an adjustment to the lens through which I saw the world. On one particular occasion I met a friend for lunch, and as the waiting staff showed us to our table, they said "This way please, ladies". There was something familiar yet new in how these words sounded. I must have been welcomed this way hundreds of times, just hearing it as the noise people make when they greet me in this environment. This time I found myself grimacing, almost physically recoiling from it. "Lady". Ugh no. There was something in it I really wanted to shake off. I felt it hemming me in, boxing and restricting me. I felt ladened with a particular kind of stereotypical femininity I don't identify with. A delicacy, a submissiveness. Something of me was lost in being identified in this way.

I was starting to see what happens when I turn the spotlight onto my experience and scrutinise it in the same way as it is expected, demanded of the trans and non-binary people I know. Firstly, I tune in to the privilege of this scrutiny being a choice. In this instance, I reflected that the word "lady" has probably always felt inaccurate for me, but it just hasn't caused enough discomfort for me to have to pay much attention. I take this for granted—the ability not to have to consider the labels I am given and the assumptions they hold, because they are at best a good fit and at worst, bearable. In examining my own response, I am able to connect to a shared human experience (e.g. being labelled), which opens up a sense of how differently this might play out for someone else. For me, the label is grating, but it is not misgendering, fundamentally invalidating or erasing. It felt uncomfortable, but not harmful, exposing or dangerous.

Secondly, recognising how gender norms and expectations can limit and restrict me personally helps confront the part of me that can hold an internalised othering attitude. It makes more visible to me the expansive freedom and beauty that is to be found beyond strict gender norms and assumptions—a beauty demonstrated by trans and non-binary people themselves. I believe it is not just trans and non-binary people who stand to benefit from highlighting and pulling apart society's fixed ideas about gender. We all have a stake in this battle. The injustice, however, is that it tends to fall on those most impacted, who feel the oppression most violently, to take it on. I am reminded here, of hearing public figure and trans activist Munroe Bergdorf speak about burnout as an activist. She described the heavy and destructive weight of the discrimination and backlash felt by trans and non-binary people in this position, and the important role cis allies can play in sharing the load, given our "broader shoulders" for issues that do not affect us.

"Is there something you need to tell us?"

Yes, it's about me and it's not about me.

I'm learning that being an ally is a dynamic state. Introspection is an important place to visit, but not a constructive place to dwell. Self-examination is proving to be a useful route to both connection with others and a greater appreciation for the stark differences in experience.

The point is, it serves a purpose. It is not self-examination for self-examination's sake. As an ally, if I don't consider my reflections in relation to those I stand beside, I risk missing the bigger picture. I was speaking with a friend about this delicate balance with introspection as an ally, and she brilliantly captured what can be at stake: "While we navel gaze, people die".

Having really come to understand the importance of acknowledging and exploring my positioning as an ally, I was frustrated to notice an old pattern coming up when preparing for this chapter. I was writing about a conversation with my husband and stopped as I saw the word "partner" appear on the screen. I stopped because it felt so unnatural for me to use this word, but something had drawn me to type it in place of "husband". I quickly recognised the old awkwardness in revealing how heteronormative I am and immediately felt frustrated. I thought I'd resolved this imposter thing! ... Ah ... "Resolved" ... A trap I was trying to avoid falling into, I reminded myself. I was learning to try to move away from rigid, binary thinking, which is where quicksand lies. To stay responsive and attuned as an ally, it's important that I remain open and curious. It's important that I am willing to revisit things, examine them from different angles and accept this as part of the messy, never ending job of navigating the world in general.

"Is there something you need to tell us?"

Yes, this is an ongoing process.

I am continually finding and revisiting parts of myself that need examining. I was recently reflecting on the fact that a number of the trans and non-binary people I know had all been speaking to me about barriers to social transition. People were describing wanting to present more authentically in the world, but feared being highlighted as different, receiving unwanted attention and facing the dangers this might bring. I noticed a barrier in myself when hearing these experiences, something making it difficult for me to meet people where they were. It was an eagerness, I wanted to rush them to the finish line. While I heard their fear, I found myself focused on wanting to help people "just get out there". I caught this as something to be examined. I was the eager one, the people speaking to me were hesitant. There was a tug of war going on within me which felt completely at odds with my way of engaging with people, trying to be alongside them in their challenges, not battling with them. So why was I positioning myself in this way? What was being played out? I wondered.

When I looked at the eagerness, I recognised a sense of the inevitability that people would need to face these fears at some stage, so the sooner they were able to acclimatise the better. "The sooner the better?" I was shocked to find this in the mix. When I played it back to myself, there was an impatience in it, a harshness even. Not to mention an assumption that people *would* or *could* acclimatise! I couldn't make sense of why I was taking such a perspective. Identifying it came as another wakeup call, alerting me to a place I was definitely imposing some of my own meaning or assumptions onto other people's experiences. I was taken back by the strength of my feeling and it took me some time to put my finger on what was motivating it.

Unsurprisingly, a strong feeling was being driven by a strongly held belief: Everyone should be able to express themselves authentically in the world. I wholeheartedly stand by this; however, something was getting lost in translation and was manifesting in a less than helpful way. I was holding onto something. But what?

There has been a powerful discourse growing in recent history about being "out and proud" about gender and sexual diversity.[3] And so there should be. But it now struck me that somewhere along the line, I had translated this into a fairly fixed assumption that "out is best". Inevitably. Always. I think I was driven by a sense of responsibility as an ally to echo and somehow reinforce this internalised belief. On one level, "out is best" does make sense, because in an ideal world there would be no need to "come out" at all, it would be meaningless. In our less-than-ideal world, however, out can be frightening, risky or explicitly unsafe. I knew

---

[3] "Gender and sexual diversity" is a term increasingly used in place of acronyms such as LGBTQIA + (Lesbian, Gay, Bisexual, Transgender, Queer, Intersex, Asexual and identities other than these). While no term can be entirely unproblematic, there are several reasons acronyms might be problematic: the inherent presentation of an order; erasing unrepresented identities; the "Alphabet Soup" effect, of endlessly extending the acronym to be as inclusive as possible leading to a cumbersome phrase for use in general parlance.

this. I had seen how this was the case for numerous people in my life but knowing it had somehow not been enough in this instance to interrupt what I had internalised. It actually makes me cringe, reflecting on what was playing out here. Here I was, as someone with no lived experience of coming out, on some level holding a sense of "knowing best" about it. How easily that colonial dynamic I was so concerned about can be at play. If my eagerness had gone unexamined, it could have been harmful. Engaging from this position would have risked alienating the people who were sharing their struggles with me, potentially invalidating experiences and even bringing additional shame where people may be already struggling with forms of internalised shame.

Having started to understand and pull apart my eagerness, I began to hear what people were saying with more clarity. I realised I had not really heard the fear at all, and now, people's words hit me with force. Fear of the spotlight. Fear of that implicitly Othering gaze. Fear of ridicule, rejection and abuse. Fear of physical violence. Hearing this with a more attuned ear, unencumbered by previous assumptions, there was something that resonated.

I found myself whisked back to my teenage years and felt the heat of a familiar spotlight penetrate my skin. As a young person in a body often labelled "fat" by others, I had a sense of there being no safe space, no escape from objectification and scrutiny. Strangers, or people I knew, could all place this spotlight on me, whether I wanted them to or not. Whether I consented or not. They would pick me out as different, unacceptable in some way. I always had the sense that whatever I did, "fat" was how people saw me first. Memories tumbled back over me with visceral weight. The feeling of being wrapped up in the heady joys of a teenage night out, the euphoric bubble of booze, music and sweaty embraces on the dancefloor, and the feeling of that bubble instantly bursting at the sound of words shouted in my direction: "It's a fat bird with a nose ring!" The same crushing feeling when I won a 100-m race in an athletics competition and a "friend" commented, "Fair play, you run pretty quick for a fat bitch".

Those old, familiar feelings hit me like a tidal wave. The knot in my stomach, the tension in my chest. The feeling of wanting to hide away and not expose myself to such scrutiny. That gaze I had experienced as unfamiliar in responding to the Facebook comment—perhaps there was something I did recognise. In sharing these memories, I do not intend to present them as overtly traumatic or equate them with the dangers faced by trans and non-binary people. I simply want to demonstrate that when I am truly present with another person and really attend to my own response, it is possible to find a powerful connection. I cannot know how it feels to navigate social transition. I can, however, find connection to the human experience of feeling observed, objectified and ostracised. I can connect to the apprehension and fear of facing this, and the far-reaching impact of learning to view myself through the same lens others have used.

"Is there something you need to tell us?"

Yes, but it's not a neat ending. Or an ending at all in fact.

In considering how to draw my reflections together, I find myself thinking "what have I learnt?" Which is interesting as this is the central point I have come to—I am, and always will be, in the process of learning. I initially considered myself positioned to be a strong ally to the trans and non-binary community, having close relationships with LGBT[4] people, a liberal viewpoint on the world and a deep sense of social justice. While these factors of course help me align myself with the trans and non-binary rights movement, there was a short-sightedness in this perspective—an assumption that this is enough, that I have ticked the boxes and earned my badge.

What I am unpacking is the importance of, or rather responsibility to keep going further than this. When I have gone further and taken a curious attitude towards myself as an ally, I have moved through many positions. Initially, there was a sense of going from one extreme to another, from feeling ideally positioned to having no position at all from which to engage. There it was again—the restrictive binary thinking. Perhaps the allure of fixed positions is the illusion that we can have things

---

[4] Language is dynamic. I have used "Gender and sexual diversity" elsewhere in the chapter to refer to a broad and diverse group, but here I use the acronym "LGBT", because "Lesbian", "Gay", "Bisexual" or "Trans" are the specific terms the particular people I am referring to use to describe themselves.

"sussed", but of course we can't. Human experience is far too awkward and messy. So how can we expect our engagement with human issues to be anything but awkward and messy? Ultimately my journey is about turning towards the messiness, and learning that when I do this, I can't clean it up, but through it I can find greater connection.

The Uncanny

At the heart of many social dilemmas and personal distress is the view of people as selfcontained rational beings. We have models that explain intellect and emotion in this way and strides are being made so that much of our economic, political and social life is moderated by mathematical models and algorithms. Even in the domain of psychotherapy, that most attuned of healing practices, the tyranny of the rational is being imposed with far more attention being given to cognitive models than the emotional and relational. Through all of this a view is promoted of an easy and straightforwardly navigated life being possible—even expected. Many of us buy into this, which makes it harder and even more confusing when we find ourselves struggling with the paradoxes of life.

Much human interaction occurs outside of awareness. Despite our intellect and technological skills, we remain instinctive, relational and embodied beings relying on long held values, emotions and practices that have served us well, over millennia. The counterintuitive and the uncanny are a part of this and are forceful influences upon our experience, our choices and our relationships—as the contributors to this final part explore.

These three chapters explore intimate, unsettling experiences of the uncanny, those moments when we feel lost, out of sorts, unsure of who we even are, or what to make of the world. They are personal accounts even when reflecting on other people or culture. Despite the personal nature, what is explored is the ephemeral, slippery nature of the uncanny and the attempts we undertake to come back from it. The experiences may not be easy to capture in language, or with any ultimate truth, but as you will see, these contributors offer useful insights, showing the informative experiences that, if reflected upon, can help us understand ourselves more fully, and maybe also the other.

Anastasios Gaitanides invites readers to explore a difficult and intimate experience—that of being bereaved. The need to find a way through an absence, a nothingness, is always hard. Anastasios courageously offers an insight into the ways in which, in bereavement, we may not only lose the person but the world as we have experienced it up to now, and how it changes, socially, emotionally and even physically. This painful experience can initially feel so bereft of meaning that we are cast adrift at a time of great need. His own process, his questioning and his openness offer the reader important reflective space.

In her chapter Elena Manafi explores the power of the the uncanny in the familiar. She explores an experience of seeing ourselves "in" the other and she explores what this means for the possibilities and problems of closer engagement. Elena writes about this very personal impact in a professional context—when she is working as a therapist, thereby exploring another limit to the "and/or" binary that so blights much human experience. The personal and the professional are not as separate as we sometimes claim.

The final chapter is my own, where I explore the power of seeing and being seen - both by self and by the other. It touches on themes in Elena's chapter and in my earlier Madame X chapter too. I explore how it is through being accurately recognised that we find a way back to ourselves and to the world. The hope is that readers will take the opportunity to think beyond the binary, and more about the relationship with themselves, with self and other and the world that we become clearer and more able to navigate the precariousness of life.

Being a Refugee in a World Without Refuge

Anastasios Gaitanidis

Waking up in the morning begins with a vague pre-reflective awareness of one's existence in the present moment. This is then followed by the recognition of current space and location—the feeling of whether one is at home or not. It is only after the "now and here" are firmly established that a sense of "I" is engendered. One's subjectivity is predicated upon the pre-reflective realisation of one's embodiment within a—often familiar—time and space.

For a long time after my wife died, I woke up but only to find myself enveloped by a shroud of yesterdays and a concatenation of vacuous tomorrows … and although I was expecting to find myself at home, I woke up instead feeling stranded into a place that bore an uncanny resemblance to a detention centre.

This was my reality, the reality of someone who is struck by grief. And the grief struck is a refugee, a migrant of love. Having lost the loved one,

---

A. Gaitanidis (✉)
Kent, UK
e-mail: anastasios.gaitanidis@rpt-ltd.co.uk

© The Author(s), under exclusive license to Springer Nature Switzerland AG 2021
M. Milton (ed.), *Balancing on Quicksand*,
https://doi.org/10.1007/978-3-030-79136-0_12

his homeland, he is forced to wander every land only to find himself arriving to a no-man's land—a place between the "not anymore" and the "not yet".

This is a surreal place, a place which is incomprehensible unless you have been struck by grief. Suddenly, stories that did not make any sense before began to make perfect sense now. I used to find bitterly funny the image of the recently bereaved old man in the animated movie *Up* who elevates his home with the aid of thousands of balloons in order to transport it to a place in South America called "Paradise Falls" because this was his wife's last wish. Lo and behold, 8 months after my wife passed away, I was on my way to South America visiting the famous "Iguazú Falls" because she wanted to go there before she died.

I could not understand how Orpheus would turn and look at Eurydice, knowing that he would lose her again, forever. Surely, no one in his "right mind" would do so… But Orpheus, like anyone who lost the person he loved the most, is quite literally "out of his mind". How many times did I catch myself saying, "If I could only see her once more, only for a brief moment, and then I could lose her again…"? How many times did I wish to catch a glimpse of her in order to feel I'm home again, only to realise that I'm not?

How can you live with the knowledge that you cannot return home anymore? For even if there is the slightest possibility of returning, the home you left behind is never the home you return to. So, how can you live with the knowledge of such a profound catastrophe?

And what does it mean to arrive? How can you arrive at, and create, another home when you have not really left the previous one behind? How do you manage to arrive somewhere, anywhere else when in your heart your final destination is actually the point of departure? How can you ever make yourself at home again without betraying the memory of the home you left behind?

Perhaps, one way to deceive yourself is to flood yourself with memories of home, to remember and hold on to everything—when you have lost so much, you don't want to lose anything else ever again, even the smallest, apparently most ordinary things. I would keep my wife's key ring and cigarette case in my pocket, it contained the last cigarette she rolled before she died. I would wear her favourite scarf over my head and nose in order to get a whiff of her lingering aroma, call her mobile repeatedly to listen to her voicemail message and write a letter to her almost every day for a whole year:

My dear wife,
"Pain" – in this single word I try to condense my upset, my disappointment, my loss.
There are times I experience pain that builds up and comes out like a torrent that destroys everything that stands on its way. There is also pain that I try to displace onto others in order to manage it from a distance.
But mostly there is pain that demands to be felt, pain that either crawls its way up through my skin or inhabits the subterranean field of expressionless rage. It is so expansive that it floods my entire relational universe. This pain simultaneously builds me up and tears me down; it both connects me with and dissociates me from you. This pain is hard, almost impossible, to bear.
But the most excruciating pain of all is the one you had experienced for such a long time, my love: relentless physical pain. It gnawed at you, repeatedly biting bits of your soul, attempting to destroy your humanity.
I am sorry. I shouldn't complain to you... I simply don't know how to handle my pain.
Your husband,
A.

And then I would reply to my letter on her behalf:

My darling husband,
There is no need to apologise. The amount of pain we experienced... I am absolutely amazed by our capacity to endure so much pain. And, yet, this pain did not make us 'ugly'. Our humanity did not evaporate under the constant assault of cancerous ignominy. We were not going to be defeated out of our dignity.
You see, my love, cancer was this ominous, dark cloud hanging over us that was trying to overshadow us. But it was constantly failing. Please remember I didn't die of cancer. Cancer died with me.
Your wife,
M.

Yet, when remembering and writing letters does not work anymore, the only other way you could fool yourself into believing that you could feel like home again is to purge yourself of any memory, to cut yourself off from anything that might remind you of your previous home. You attempt to forget… you don't talk about it. This is certainly what my refugee parents tried to do. They remained silent about the pain of their forced displacement. And, in any case, even when they felt the need to talk about it, nobody wanted to listen—this could have been interpreted as being "negative" or not trusting the possibility of creating a life in their new homeland. But, you see, that's the thing about pain: it is noisy—it demands our attention, especially when we try to bury it underneath multiple layers of silence. It is not an accident therefore that the unearthing of traumas has become my vocation.

It was my attempt to break through this silence—and, perhaps, reconnect with the pain of my parents—that made me visit their homeland during the summer of 2016 only to find myself, by a bizarre coincidence or a weird twist of fate, in the middle of a military coup. "Is it possible in this day and age for a country to have a coup?" I asked my friend, exhibiting my naivety and ignorance. "Of course, it is…", he said, "What did you expect to find by visiting this country?" To be frank, I had a lot of expectations from that visit, but I never expected to find myself in the middle of the same dangerous situation that my parents experienced 60 years ago, fearing for my life and wanting to flee the country as they did! It was almost comical in an uncanny, cruel kind of way. I guess Marx was right after all—history does repeat itself: the first time as a tragedy, the second time as a farce.[1]

And it is part of the same history that I, the son of refugees, sought refuge in another land, a British one, one that I thought exhibited the generosity of welcome that my country of origin wouldn't and couldn't exhibit. And for a while (25 years) this seemed to be working: I felt at home—I loved my work, I loved my wife, I loved this country. And then, the woman I so dearly loved was no longer alive and the country I used to believe in was gradually, *Brexitically*, disappearing. The only thing left

---

[1] Marx (1852).

was my work as a therapist, the refuge I provided for all the walking wounded that came to see me.

When I began my training as a psychoanalytic therapist, I was 27. I had a placement with a charity organisation that provided support and counselling for carers of partners, spouses, friends or relatives who suffered a variety of chronic physical and mental illnesses. I had seen husbands caring for their ailing wives, brothers for their siblings, mothers and fathers for their sons and daughters.

I distinctly remember working with a man in his late 50s who was forced to take early retirement in order to look after his epileptic wife, only to lose her a year later after having a massive epileptic fit and stroke. He was inconsolable. I could barely stay with his despair and loneliness wondering what I could possible "do" for him in sixteen sessions. It was November 1997; we finished therapy in March 1998. In the last session, I was curious to find out whether I did anything that made a difference to his life. He replied: "You helped me get through the winter". Eighteen years later, I would utter the exact same words to my therapist, realising that the best thing she "did" for me during the year following my wife's death was to provide me with a "talking shelter" and have the courage to witness my raw, unformulated pain.

Is therapy the only place that could conjure up an image of home? Surely not. There must be other places, other refuges that can summon into existence the idea of home. Well, I'm not so sure anymore. The few places that used to provide a safety net for those unfortunate enough to be cast adrift by the nightmarish vicissitudes of life, politics and history are starting to dwindle. And what is worse, most people who have experienced these nightmares, who have lost their homes, language, spouses, relatives and friends, "choose" to forget this history, to forget all the things that have previously made their lives meaningful because, in the new homeland in which they now live, no one wants to know and share their grief. This could be "uncomfortable"—and grief is very uncomfortable, especially another person's grief.

We tend therefore to reduce the grief and pain of the other to a form of private property instead of seeing it as what underpins one's very existence and identity. For our grief and pain reveal not only that we are constituted but are also undone by our relations to others and places.

When we lose the loved one (whether a person or a place), we lose more than their luminous presence; we lose some-*one* or some-*thing* inside us that could not be replaced with anyone or anything else. Not even their memory could provide a consoling substitute for their unique existence. There is this "surplus" in every significant loss which cannot be accounted for and which is simultaneously constitutive and unsettling of our sense of self. For when we lose the person, or place, we love (our home), our anchoring points disappear, we become unmoored and drift away, like a boat or a kite in the middle of a hurricane. What we need is a port in the storm, a community (a world) whose members are aware of the "vulnerable" relational web of their grievable lives.[2] What we need is an open door, a glass of wine and a place on the table for the grieving other, the stranger, the stateless exile subject to the cruel gaze of the state. What we need is to start the conversation with this stranger who is, after all, part of ourselves…

References

Butler, J. (2009). *Frames of war: When is life grievable?* Verso Books.
Marx, C. (1963 [1852]). *The eighteenth brumaire of Luis Bonaparte.* International Publishers.

---

[2] Butler (2009).

An Uncanny Resemblance

Elena Manafi

"There are people who feel that the world is their oyster and others who wish they had never been born at all. I belong to the latter; I am in mourning for my life".[1] That is how she introduced herself to me 10 years ago. The words were uttered with a calm, composed voice while looking at me straight in the eyes with an air of defiance that filled me with warmth and trepidation. She walked into my consulting room dressed all in black; shades still on her head, unveiling her dark green eyes and the smoky make up. I knew nothing about her. She was an urgent referral from a friend and colleague of mine, who cryptically said *Manafi, this one is for you*. Little did I know back then… I was in for a ride and to this date when I think of our work together, I am filled with gratitude and humbleness.

---

[1] "I am in mourning for my life" Paraphrasing the opening lines of Chekov's play *The Seagull*.

E. Manafi (✉)
London, UK

I have always been attracted to philosophy and the arts; in my teens and throughout my early 20s—before life set out a course for me to become a psychotherapist—I spent a lot of time immersed in reading and writing—mostly diaries that kept me sane. My outlook in living was inevitably shaped by literary characters who were grappling with the human condition and the legacy of a cultural heritage that weighed heavy on my shoulders. I am still suspicious of any light that denies its shadow and of any belief that shies away from despair. Essentially, I am suspicious of all binary oppositions and can only find solace in paradoxical perspectives that embrace polarities and leave the margin of the unknown intact. I feel comfortable with contradictions. Ambiguity, abstractions, absurdity and metaphors fill me with a sense of freedom till angst and dread envelop me and force me to find a ground that provides enough certainty for me to walk on. I am an only child and can live in my head comfortably—enough to come across as a solipsist at times, but I also grew up with dogs that gave me an immense love for nature, adventure and for anything that involves physicality. In the eyes of those who know me well enough, I am a *walking contradiction* that forever tries to balance itself. I am also a psychotherapist who—to this date—finds it difficult to define what this profession is all about. What I do know from experience though is that we cannot "escape" ourselves and that all that we are accompanies us in the consulting room. So, in my view, it is imperative to get to know ourselves as much as possible so that when with an "Other",[2] we can be present in the fullest possible way without imposing but also without concealing our being. It is a fragile balancing act that can never be fully accomplished and so requires courage and strength at the face of an inherent uncertainty which results in a sense of inadequacy and vulnerability. Indeed, our capacity to tolerate vulnerability, uncertainty and the anxiety they provoke is at the heart of our practice.

I have spent many years trying to create for myself a psychotherapeutic perspective that incorporates the wisdom I found in philosophy and the arts as well as the wider socio-political, cultural, and historical context within which we are all embedded. Gradually, I drifted away from approaches that attempt to control, predict, quantify and

---

[2] Capital "O" is intentional to affirm difference and otherness.

explain the irreducible experience of Being[3] and have come to understand that becoming a therapist necessitates an embodied awareness of our modes of understanding the world and others. It is our personal and professional responsibility to question our assumptions about human beings and the world we live in, as well as, the premises that underly our efforts to explore and investigate the human condition and our clients' predicament in particular. In the words of Willig, we need to develop "ontological and epistemological reflexivity[4]". The ontological premises that underly my engagement with the world on both personal and professional levels place conflict, anguish, despair, disillusionment and loss at its centre. I view human beings as a synthesis of opposites—capable of "taking stock" and reflecting upon themselves, others, the world and their mode of conduct. I also believe that self-deception is at the heart of our being and in many ways the greatest defence against anguish and pain. This ability to "stand out" and reflect upon our existence comes with a price as it creates a fundamental sense of lack in our being which leaves us always yearning for completion. We are embedded and embodied, condemned to meaning and choice, and we are also subject to forces (both internal and external) that lie outside our control. In essence, the "deliberate I"—this cherished subjectivity of ours—is inextricably linked to the "Other", our "situatedness" (i.e., culture, history, society, class, race, political and socio-economic status), and the influence of powerful ideologies that create the illusion of permanence and security. Navigation in such a complex landscape is a constant struggle; self-deception becomes unavoidable as it helps to avoid pain, vulnerability, and most importantly responsibility and the anxiety inherent in the human condition.

D.[5] was a white, Italian woman, in her mid-30s—a solemn figure with a loud laughter that occasionally filled the room with promise and lightness in the midst of her pain and her sense of doom. By the end of our first session, I had a good sense why *The Seagull* had come to mind. Her

---

[3] Capital "B" is also intentional to denote existence (the human condition in the broadest sense of the word).

[4] Willig (2019, p. 186).

[5] All personal information has been changed to ensure my client's anonymity and secure confidentiality.

longing for freedom and carefree security had been repeatedly crashed at the hands of a loved one, her mother. Lost in the maze of a tempestuous childhood and upbringing, she was left feeling trapped, torn and heavy. Her lived experience is best captured by a recurring dream that she often brought to our sessions to haunt us and that confirmed—in her mind— that life is elsewhere, that it never belonged to her and that it never will. The dream represented the actuality of her experience in the moment, in the "now" where the past merged with the present and brought with it the painful recognition that her past had not passed at all. Indeed, the dream captured the narrative of her entire life.

> *It's dusk. I am running away from a burning house. I am exhausted and covered with blood, but I keep running, repeating to myself "don't look back, don't look back". Ahead of me a green field. I can sense the freedom and desire. I can see a shelter that I desperately try to reach. Suddenly, I hear a voice. It's my mother, I turn and look. She is emerging from the flames and I freeze.*

It was not D's darkness that petrified me, but our uncanny resemblance.

We shared a passion for the arts and philosophy; many literary and artistic "giants" kept us company during our sessions. Dostoyevsky, Tolstoy, Schopenhauer, Nietzsche, Baldwin, Beckett, Bergman, Almodóvar, Kundera, Woody Allen (when in the mood for a joke) and pretty much all the novels and plays written by existential thinkers like Sartre, Camus and de Beauvoir. They all became silent companions to our gradual decent into the despair of her abyss. Like *fellow sufferers*[6] (a greeting that resonated with both of us), they offered consolation, clarity and courage in her attempts to confront her pain and the limitations and contingency of the human condition. They became a torch in her efforts to create a niche in a world that often felt "upside down" and in her struggle to negotiate the tension between polarities that are quintessentially human: relatedness and alienation; enmeshment and separation; intimacy and autonomy; strength and vulnerability; recognition and

---

[6] Schopenhauer's greeting to fellow human beings.

negation; belonging and isolation; freedom and determinism; order and chaos.

I faced a number of dilemmas in our work together; upon reflection, I cannot fail to notice that all of them emerged out of my immediate encounter with her in our sessions (i.e. interpersonal dimension) as well as my encounter with myself—or rather, to be more precise with who I thought I was! My desire is to communicate my learning from this encounter, which I hope will be of use to others. I will avoid referencing (unless I am using a quote) established knowledge and instead stay with my own reflections and feelings. This is not because I don't see value in research and the academia in general—after all my personal is always *in relation* to what exists (or not) out there—but because I want to pay tribute to the exposure I felt and to my client's voice[7] in the absence of the (illusionary) security "evidence" provides. This is an invitation to ponder, feel, think and reflect with me.

For me to be able to be of any use to my clients, I need to retain *"one foot in and one foot out"* as I often say to my students. This stance is vital and for the sake of both of us: "the foot in" acknowledges and embraces both of our subjectivities in the room and gives me—the therapist—the opportunity to reflect upon my being (in holistic terms) in relation to my client. It allows me to consider what I bring (or not) to the session and why; to use my therapeutic knowledge and skills at the service of my client and to reflect upon my affectivity—meaning my "how" in the session. This "how" includes my reactions, attitudes, feelings, values, thoughts and everything that informs my stance and interventions. I rely upon this "foot" as it sustains not only my attunement to my client's emotional world, but also my awareness of the ways in which I am being affected by the issues explored and his/her predicament as a whole. The "foot out" is of equal importance and a clarification is necessary here: "out" does not imply objectivity (I have lost faith in this word a long time ago) but the preservation of Otherness while still in relation. This "foot" collaborates with the client and attempts to make sense of the latter's

---

[7] This reflective piece is a purposeful elaboration of my work with an actual client who has given consent for the material used.

lived experience. It enables me to observe what is happening within my client, between us and within me.

The questions I kept asking myself were "how *actual* can I be without impeding upon the therapeutic process?"[8] "have I sufficiently confronted my own demons or will they come back to haunt me, rendering me incapable to "walk" side by side with my client (rather than ahead)?" "Will I be able to tune in to her experience without imposing my being and without misrepresenting her pain?" Such questions made me vigilant throughout my work with D. and brought to the surface my silent confrontation with the person I thought I was. It turned out that my attunement to her activated my own past, my own struggles and desires and most importantly my own defences. Our "uncanny resemblance" often paralysed me, leaving me experiencing intense emotions and at times an inability to distinguish what was mine and what was hers. Losing the safety of Otherness—the previously thought clear line of demarcation between me and her—was not easy to navigate. Without any volition on my part, I was often transported to my childhood, replaying memories and dramas in my mind, that filled me with suspicion as I was no longer sure whose experience I was understanding and reflecting upon: hers, mine or an amalgamation of both?

The more I was tuning in, the more passionate I was becoming, blinded by my own needs, convictions and desire to "save" my client from the traps I had fallen in and from the "doomness" that stopped her from living. In the absence of personal therapy and supervision, I wouldn't have realised that I had turned into a flamingo that was standing on one foot (the one within) with defiance—ready to obliterate any obstacles standing in the way of our work together! I am now laughing at the face of my omnipotence, this trickster that filled me with a sense of power when in reality, I was shit-scared, vulnerable and at the mercy of powerful enactments. Power! We take pride in our profession and its emphasis on equality and empowerment and yet we rarely stop to reflect upon what motivated us to become therapists in the first

---

[8] I strongly recommend to the reader Hans Cohn's (1989) brilliant paper on "The place of the Actual in Psychotherapy"— it's a rare combination of personal reflections and psychotherapeutic theory.

place. Who had I become? Plenty of powerful positions to choose from—the combination that described me best is that of a wounded healer, riding to the rescue, ready to stand by my client through thick and thin and possibly fall off the cliff together! The glory of self-deception had triumphantly entered the consulting room and—to repeat—if it wasn't for personal therapy and supervision, I would have fallen flat on my face. Power is inherent in all human relations but, especially in the one between therapist and client hence the emphasis on standards, ethics, professional conduct etc. What if, however, all this becomes a cover? Learning about power and its abusive potential is one thing, experiencing it is quite another. Finding out who we become at the face of power necessitates personal reflection and examination of our motivations and function of defences. This cannot be done through reading; this, can only be done though experiencing what it feels and means to be a client ourselves. I was lucky to complete trainings that fully valued the role of personal therapy, supervision, reflexivity and experiential work and that were suspicious of words such as "expertise", "authority" and "certainty", and yet (clearly) luck was not enough which makes me respect the power of self-deception even more and the value of self-examination, especially when we feel on top of our game!

It was the painstaking recognition of my enmeshment with my client that brought me back to my senses and allowed me to slowly reclaim the necessary stance of "negative capability[9]" that deprived me of my memory, desire and understanding and allowed me to regain my own equanimity, become receptive, and practice the ethics of ambiguity, tolerance and uncertainty. Only then was I able to create space for my client's experience to emerge and find its own home. My analyst and my supervisor once again became my torch; the former held me in my abyss and helped me confront the residues of my past experience. The latter reminded me that "what is familiar and well known as such is not really known for the very reason that it is *familiar and well known*[10] ".

---

[9] Rollins (2012).
[10] Hegel (2019, p. 20). Emphasis in the original.

I realised that our uncanny resemblance was not the ally I thought it was. My identification with D. veiled my understanding of her experience and led to premature interpretations and consolidation of meaning. D had become my "imaginary twin" and Bion was spot on in thinking that "the function of the imaginary twin is to deny a reality different from [our own][11]". I am pretty sure that I was compensating for all the years I spent alone trying to comprehend my reality; in many ways it facilitated the development of a strong bond with D., but it also killed my curiosity and blurred the line of demarcation that separated us. Through my work with her, I learnt that I had to discard all that was known; to make room for silence and leave space for her thoughts, ideas and desires to disclose themselves in their own time and in their initial unintelligibility. I also learnt that if we are to dive into another person's abyss—to apprehend the inaccessible—we need to be able to wait, tolerate frustration and ambiguity and learn to listen afresh, because *how* we listen determines *what* can be heard and what is responded to.

We worked together for five years; in times of crises we would meet twice, sometimes three times a week. The increase in frequency paradoxically meant "doing" less rather than more. It was a shift that at first felt counterintuitive, as we were both caught up in a sense of urgency that kept placing demands on our work—a desire for change mostly. I soon realised that "change" has many faces—she rarely looks like what we first imagined. Change, choice, freedom, insight and so many other cherished concepts, are fiercely dynamic in nature and maybe that's why they are so difficult to be achieved. In theory—after some time—everything becomes clear, so clear that often our clients say "I know what I need to do, who I need to be, but I can't bring myself to do/be it" and so everything becomes stilted with intellectual clarity on one hand, embodied paralysis on the other and a good dose of shame and a smell of defeat in the air. That's when the good old saying "trust the process" becomes painfully pertinent. Trust the process and endure the stuckness, I may add. Easier said than done, but in my experience, that's the work during this phase of therapy: endurance and faith. Any premature moves driven by the intellectual clarity are destined to fail. That's what

---

[11] Bion (1967, p. 19).

happened with D. and myself at different stages in life—jerky movements full of passion, promises to oneself uttered with conviction, oceans of tears filled with anger and pain that dried too quickly, followed by more promises and further moves only to return to the exact same place with the exact same dream shattering the hopes of the day before. In the absence of courage (this time by the therapist) to stay with his/her own vulnerability, despair and feelings of not being good enough, the work runs the risk of becoming homework—a series of mandates that sustain the illusion of control. I am afraid there is no way out of the despair—the only way is through. The words, frequently attributed to Winston Churchill come to mind: "If you are going through hell, keep going[12]" and of Samuel Beckett, "Ever tried, ever failed. No matter. Try again. Fail again. Fail better[13]". That's how endurance and faith look and feel like in the abyss of despair.

So, we kept going, and going, and it felt endless; art (the aforementioned literary "giants", poets and screenwriters) became the only solace and consolation, because art is merciful and liberating in its transgression. It is a busy, two-way street as it expresses and satisfies the psychic needs of both artist and recipient. Art is a *catharsis* according to Aristotle (though to be fair he was referring to tragedy mostly!) and later Freud; it is the space where the imaginary and the real meet and reconcile in the most creative ways. The therapeutic use of art is invaluable because when art is explored with conscious awareness, the aforementioned intellectual insight that was so copiously gained is felt in the body like a punch in the stomach. All of a sudden, the stuckness takes a very different meaning: what was previously thought of as a passive and powerless stance now feels like an active form of avoidance. The avoidance of living the very life we always wished for and dreamt of. Those of us who feel attracted to existential thought tend to embrace the concept of death anxiety as a given, but the more I live and the more I practice, I begin to see why Jaspers[14] argued that the anxiety is not of death but of life and living.

---

[12] Although frequently attributed to Winston Churchill, it is hard to find any formal, verified reference.

[13] Beckett (1983, p. 7).

[14] For a concise secondary source on Jaspers refer to Stanghellini and Fuchs (2013).

When the punch is felt, words and thoughts are no longer necessary; their purpose has been served, the path has been paved, and the time has come to walk the talk. What is most humbling in that moment is that the move no longer requires promises to oneself, reminders and any form of effort. The move is so embodied that it cannot be stopped, it just is. The chasm that separated the polarities of existence and the ones held within is bridged and the move is performed on the tension their integration has created. What perhaps is also unavoidable is a sense of bitter/sweet melancholy that accompanies the walk as we wave goodbye to all the illusions previously held, to everything previously thought, to the sense of self previously embraced and while staring at the horizon we feel "determined to save the only life that you could save[15]".

References

Beckett, S. (1983). *Westword Ho!* John Calder.
Bion, W. R. (1967). *Second thoughts: Selected papers on psycho-analysis.* Jason Aronson.
Cohn, H. (1989). The place of actuality in psychotherapy. *Free Associations, 18,* 49–61.
Hegel, G. W. F. (2019 [1807]). *The phenomenology of spirit.* Cambridge University Press.
Oliver, M. (1986). *Dream work.* Atlantic Monthly Press
Rollins, H. E. (2012). *The letters of John Keats: 1814–1821.* Cambridge University Press.
Stanghellini, G., & Fuchs, T. (2013). *One century of Karl Jaspers' general psychopathology.* Oxford University Press.
Willig, C. (2019). Ontological and epistemological reflexivity: A core skill for therapists. *Counselling and Psychotherapy Research, 19,* 186–194.

---

[15] Oliver (1986, p. 39). In *The Journey.*

Making the Invisible Visible

Martin Milton

Tears—even a single tear—can indicate many things—despair, fear, sadness, joy among them. Tears are my "go to" reaction in the face of something powerful and meaningful. Especially something greater than words. Take these three examples …

Scene 1: David is standing by the counter. I see his face start to redden and to crumple as his partner, Patrick, sings to him. His eyes water—as do mine. Despite watching from afar, I *feel* the intensity of his emotion as a constriction in my chest. It is rich and complicated, combining pleasure and pride, an element of embarrassment, as well as delight. I wipe away the tear that flows from my eye. Then I chuckle, amazed at how I can feel so many things at once.

Scene 2: Nicholas reflects on his past, saying "I am gay. Gay - this word and everything it stands for - is what I am at the age of nine, although I have not even heard of it yet. I know it, I feel it and, in

---

M. Milton (✉)
Regent's University London, London, UK
e-mail: miltonm@regents.ac.uk

secret, I start living it". As these words register, I feel a wave of emotion, maybe the fear he experienced, the shame he had to navigate and also his determination. My own heart is sore and I have to take a breath and wipe my eyes again.

Scene 3: Last year I sat there, porous, powerless to quell the breach of the bodily boundary. I cried in relation to Toby's trauma, I cried as Eric and Jasper's friendship fell apart and I wept copiously hearing Walter trying to explain how it things were at the height of the first pandemic. At first, Eric didn't get it—he couldn't get it. So Walter asked him to tell him the name of one of his closest friends. Their conversation broke me.

Eric: Tristan.
Walter: Imagine that Tristan is dead. Name another.
Eric: Jasper.
Walter: Jasper is also dead.
Eric: Jason.
Walter: Jason has been at St Vincent's for two weeks. The toxoplasmosis has left him with dementia.
Eric: Jason, his husband.
Walter: Because they cannot legally be married, abandonment is simpler. Jason has left him.
Young Men: Patrick is dead. Alex is dead. Colin is dead. Lucas is infected. Zach is dying from Pneumocystis carinii. Chris is healthy. His partner has just been diagnosed. You just visited Mark in the hospital. Tonight you will visit Will. Tomorrow is Eddie's funeral. Michael's body is covered with KS lesions. Jeffrey is infected but asymptomatic. Nick is dead. Daniel is dead. Stephen is infected. Brian's partner has peripheral neuropathy. He screams in pain at the slightest touch. Scott is in Paris, hoping to get HPA-23. Javier went home to die in his mother's house. Jonathan's family won't take him back. Brandon is dead. Matthew is dead. Leo is infected. Kurt is infected but he doesn't know it. David, his partner, will find out first. Frankie's sister calls you to tell you he's died. Andrew has disappeared altogether. Phillip is dead. Trevor is dead. Kevin is infected. Rumours fly about incarcerations of gay men as a precaution. Politicians begin to openly discuss mass quarantines. There is talk of outlawing homosexuality, rumours of deportations. Anti-gay violence is on the rise. The American public becomes galvanised by the epidemic: not against the illness but against the people who have it.

Businesses cancel health insurance policies for employees with AIDS. States pass legislation requiring home sellers to divulge if a person with AIDS has ever lived there. Sam is dead. Mark is dead. Miguel is infected. Paul has it. Ben has it. Carlos has it. Wesley is dead. Caleb is dead. David is dead. Jacob is dead.
Walter: That is what it was.

This tsunami of disaster had me defenceless, hit by one loss after another, each one a devastating blow. If I had been standing, I would have collapsed. The pain was visceral and immense.

I cried even though my involvement in these experiences was not straightforward. In some ways, you could say that I was not actually involved. Not as a full participant, not like when I held our beloved Jordan for the vet to administer the final, merciful escape. I was not physically in the room to be so moved by David and Patrick—I couldn't be, *Schitt's Creek* is filmed in Canada, and I was watching during the first lockdown in London. While Nicholas' words felt like the most intimate of disclosures, I was reading Andre Carl van der Merwe's[1] novel tucked up at home. And while I was technically in the room with Toby, Eric and Walter, I was separate, safely perched on my theatre seat as Andy Burnap, Kyle Soller and Paul Hilton performed in Mathew Lopez's outstanding play, *The Inheritance*.[2]

I am a therapist by trade, someone entrusted with real people's pain and struggle on a regular basis and so am somewhat used to feeling emotion. While some forms of therapy aim primarily for intellectual clarity, when psychotherapy works best, an attentive, attuned therapist is invested in *seeing* you as fully and authentically as possible. I know this from my work and from my experience as a client too. My therapists have helped me face what I could not bear to imagine—loss, fear and panic. With those experiences, I understand when people argue that therapy is—can be? Should be?—something deep and important and that comparatively theatre and storytelling are just that—stories. Art? Entertainment maybe?

---

[1] Van der Merwe (2011).
[2] Lopez (2018, pp. 62–64).

Yet I don't buy that. On the contrary, the more I immerse myself in my work, and also in storytelling, the more I see the parallels. They are all ways of co-inhabiting personal experience. When you connect—whether in the consulting room, or through art—it is profoundly powerful.

It is this power that means on occasion, I have not been able to keep my experiences to myself. Tears are one visible manifestation of what these moments meant to me. So was my writing. I wrote about *Moffie* in *The Psychologist*.[3] Likewise, *The Inheritance*,[4] I raved about it to anyone that would let me. I talked about the words, I marvelled at the acting. I shared how affected I was with Kyle Soller's mind-blowing performance—those long, emotionally complex speeches. Soller was on stage for a huge part of the 7 hours it played out. Andy Burnap's stark, high energy, over the top delight and plunges into deep despair took me with him. How is it that something passive, "watching" something, could leave me so exhausted?

Art is art and is always being reviewed, debated and its value contested. The pandemic has, once again, asked us to think about our relationship with it. Its value is brought front and centre as theatres and cinemas have closed, book festivals have had to go online and the British government told dancers and other creatives to retrain—in cyber. A thoughtless, dismissive downgrading of the place of art, a failure to recognise its place in a psychologically healthy society.[5]

As I said, I am a therapist, I am not an artist, nor an art historian. I have stood in front of some of the most celebrated pieces—in front of a Venetian Tintoretto I appreciated the colours but was I moved? Not really. While others whispered in awe in front of the Mona Lisa I thought "Is that it?" And Pinter plays? I just can't be doing with them. Actors may rave, but I am bored, annoyed by the dated content, and the brown and beige that seems to colour every set.

---

[3] Milton (2014).

[4] Milton (2018, 2019).

[5] Neither neoliberalism nor the economic damage of a pandemic should mean that we turn to economics alone. If we are to survive well—personally and culturally—we have to think about the ways in which we are seen and understood, how we tell our own stories—whether that is within our families, to therapists or within the cogs of the neoliberal economic machine that runs much of our world.

Art brings forth a diversity of experience. I was blown away by *The Inheritance*, a close friend of mine wasn't. We thought it through. It took a while as it wasn't an easy, straightforward assessment of some "objective" quality. It wasn't that one of us had misunderstood the meaning of theatre, we hadn't made a mistake in assessing the acting, or scoring the script. For us, the key difference was that I saw *my* life up there, captured, cared for and beautifully attended to. While she "got" that, appreciated it, learnt something and thought it worthy—there was nothing of her story up there. She missed seeing women. She missed having storylines she could identify with. As I felt central, she felt excluded.

Art is powerful, as are our responses to it. They remind us of our uniqueness, our solitariness, our distinctiveness. Is that any different to therapy? To medicine? Or citizenship? None of these will be experienced in one single, generic way.

But like these, art is important. The possibility of making a person feel—whether they were prepared to or not—is an important part of the artistic endeavour. Its ability to communicate something meaningful is central. Stories—whether televised, on the pages of a novel or up there on stage—can touch us in extraordinarily powerful ways. They speak to people, reflecting lives across time and place. It is about attunement despite our differences and it is primal.

Art is storytelling and storytelling is a personal, psychological and spiritual endeavour. Stories allow us to be seen, and to feel understood. They can rescue us from being invisible, from being cast aside and forgotten. It is powerful to see ourselves recognised and represented in the minds of others. This may be particularly relevant for those of us who have reason not to take acceptance for granted, whose experiences and identities are rejected, stigmatised and made invisible. Lives that are tentative, precarious and for many, perpetually uncanny.

In so many ways, we see ourselves through the eyes of the other. If we are lucky, friends, lovers, and family shape our sense of who we are positively. Art too confirms our existence, our right to exist. Through this we see our pain understood, our fears held in the secure space of a stage or the close-able pages of a novel. Representation wards off the invisibilising, the gaslighting and the constant judgement so prevalent in our distress. For a moment they fade away. An individual can take respite here.

Being seen in this way can be life-saving—Matt Haig described reading as a "route out of yourself", or art being a way to keep ourselves sane[6]; Philip Pullman,[7] reclaiming a phrase made famous by warmongering politicians, talks of the power story has to reach both hearts and minds (2017). Agreeing that storytelling is an effective political tool, Jane Goodall has long argued that stories have a role at the level of global environmental policy. "My way is to tell stories, trying to reach the heart" she says.[8] There is power in telling stories, a power that the communication of facts alone can struggle to convey.

Art also helps us cross boundaries. *The Inheritance* and *Moffie* are set in very different places—the height of the AIDS epidemic in New York and Apartheid South Africa, but they had a similar effect on me. Maybe that is because they are both places I have lived and have a huge affection for. But it's not that straightforward, I came to *Schitts Creek* with far less identification—I have only just watched it, as an adult, and as an adult that has never been to Canada—yet it still offers experiences I identify with. I too grew up in a small (although not *that* small), conservative town where it was too easy to stand out. My identification isn't just with an individual character, but with places, with the worlds that have to be navigated.

Powerful stories capture life—in these examples, lives I anticipated but managed to escape, at least to some degree. Unlike Nicholas van der Swart, I escaped conscription into the South African army. But exile came with great costs. Unlike Walter's litany of loss, I survived the worst of the pandemic that so devastated my queer forebears, but the isolation took a toll too. Seeing these worlds writ large offers a chance to reflect in new and creative ways—to get to know the scared youngster I was,

---

[6] Guest (2017). "Haig is adamant that "one of the uses of the arts is to keep us sane", and that "reading is a route out of yourself". He is almost evangelical about the power of reading to do good. "I think books can save us and I think they sort of saved me", he says. "Empathising isn't just good for the person you're empathising with; it's good for yourself because it's a way of getting perspective over your own life. You're not the only person that matters in the world, and books are a great way of teaching yourself that".

[7] Pullman (2017).

[8] Watts (2021).

the lonely teen who wondered if he would ever find love, and in David's story, the man who has experienced the joy of being loved.

And this is another important point. Art allows us, shows us and facilitates a more imaginative set of possibilities to our dilemmas. While these stories capture the difficult aspects of life, they also champion love. Those with contested identities—queer folk growing up in heterosexist cultures, people of colour struggling in systems rooted in white supremacy, or disabled people facing the hurdles an ablest society determinedly erects, among others—are not only overlooked, but taught they are shameful, unlovable; Those are the messages we are faced with.

When I was growing up there was NO representation of men loving. Not simply an absence of gay love, but an expectation that men would demonstrate love, not through emotion or physicality but through stoic responsibility. A constant work ethic for the family was enough. So hard for straight men but for a young gay teen there was NO hope for love. Zilch. Nada. And while there was very little representation at all, that invisibility came with a quiet, audible, threatening growl.

For psychological—and social—health people need some degree of attunement from others. Being seen is crucial, knowing we are seen is important too. In families, these are the roles that we hope parents, siblings and in-laws play, culturally it is our novelists and playwrights who capture and chronicle existence, whether it be the good or bad, the knotty or straightforward. These storytellers model imaginative and creative practice, and in doing so they allow us to reflect upon ourselves, grasp our potential and understand our dilemmas. Individual and social health is on a slippery slope to nowhere if all our dancers retrain.

Most recently my tears started during the last ever episode of *Schitt's Creek*. (Spoiler—look away now if you have yet to watch it). The episode captured another of my experiences, not a life I escaped, not a period of trauma either. On this occasion, I was transported back 15 years to the day I married my husband, standing there in front of friends and family. Like David, my tears flowed. Like him, I was powerless to stop them. It was not a straightforward foreshadowing though as David limited his crying to the wedding. I continued to wipe away tears as I hugged my parents, as I took delight in seeing friends from near and far and listened to the speeches. It was wonderful. This time it was about the joy experienced when truly being seen and understood and supported. And for all this to be shared publicly.

So storytelling is not just entertainment. It is representation, it is affirmation and it is oxygen to the soul. It brings an immensely important feelings to my heart. Representation is not simply an intellectual pursuit, or a policy decision, it is emotionally woven into the fabric of community. It seems to me, that for social animals like us, storytelling is crucial. Stories bond us. It's what makes the invisible visible and helps make life worth living.

References

Guest, K. (2017, June 30). Interview: Matt Haig: 'I think books can save us: They sort of saved me'. *The Guardian.* https://www.theguardian.com/books/2017/jun/30/matt-haig-interview-books-saved-me. Downloaded 3 January 2021.

Lopez, M. (2018). *The inheritance* (pp. 62–64). Faber and Faber.

Milton, M. (2014). Moffie. *The Psychologist, 27*(1), 28–29.

Milton, M. (2018). Magical, disturbing, funny and glorious: A review of The Inheritance. *The Psychologist* (p. 55). ISSN 0952–8229.

Milton, M. (2019). The Inheritance: Reflections on visibility, representation and community wellbeing. *Psychology of Sexualities Review, 10*(1), 58–67.

Pullman, P. (2017). *Daemon voices: Essays in storytelling.* David Finckling Books.

Van der Merwe, A. C. (2011). *Moffie,* Europa.

Watts, J. (2021, January 3). Interview: Jane Goodall: 'Change is happening. There are many ways to start moving in the right way'. *The Guardian.* https://www.theguardian.com/environment/2021/jan/03/jane-goodall-change-is-happening-there-are-many-ways-to-start-moving-in-the-right-way. Downloaded 7 August 2021.

And Finally …

Martin Milton

The contributors to this volume have confirmed the experience that so many have, of life being precarious, akin to balancing on quicksand, while making profound decisions as to one's personal and social survival. We might extract ourselves and move on from any singular moment, but there is no guarantee we won't find ourselves in other equally difficult circumstances again. And again.

Throughout this volume, we have seen the value of sticking at it, trusting that slow, methodical reflection, engagement with self and other and navigating step by step, we can often thrive. We have also heard that to attune ourselves to this process, it is useful to be aware of some of the traps our psychology and cultures put in our way—such as an over-reliance on binary ways of thinking and rationality, and of utilising power without thinking about the abuses that can be so disastrous.

But the contributors have also shown how relationality helps us confront and resist the dangers we face. It helps to think of us embedded in a web of wider relationships. The more we can be curious about this ecology of relationality, the more we might understand the impact we—and our systems—have on the wider community. This in turn can contribute to greater confidence as we progress through the sticky, ever-shifting terrain we inhabit.

At least we hope so. We also hope that the ideas explored in this volume will be of use to readers in their own deliberations and as they put foot in front of foot in their efforts towards personal and cultural health and social justice.

Index

A

Activism/activist 38, 82, 87, 88, 130
Addiction 21, 22
Aggression 14, 18, 19, 118
Aguilera, Christina 111
AIDS 3, 119, 157
  epidemic 160
Ally 126–132, 134, 152
Animals 1, 34, 59, 60, 62–73, 110, 162
Antidepressants 21
Anxiety 15, 16, 22, 25, 30, 42, 70, 88, 99, 119, 146, 147, 153
Apartheid 160
Art/s 6, 38, 44, 57, 146, 148, 153, 157–161
Assessment 31, 52, 53, 56, 159
Austerity 22, 42, 87
Authority 5, 15, 17, 43, 151

B

Baldwin, James 21, 37, 39, 148
Beckett, Samuel 148, 153
Beliefs 5, 14, 62, 66, 105, 132, 146
  religious 60
Bereavement 22, 27, 86
Binary
  categories 82, 125
  oppositions 146
  thinking 3, 6, 131, 134, 163
Bipolar
  disorder 16
Black Lives Matter (BLM) 13, 81, 128
Boundary
  therapeutic 26, 27, 34
  transgression 26, 28, 31
  violation 27, 28
Brown, Brene 113
Bully/bullying 3, 22, 117, 118

Burnap, Andy 157, 158

C
Capital
   capitalism 87, 97
   punishment 50
   social 81, 84
Church 14, 17, 105
Churchill, Winston 153
Civil rights 81, 82, 120
Climate
   and ecological emergency 22
   change 1, 59, 72, 89
Cognitive
   behavioural therapy (CBT) 52
   dissonance 51
Colonialism 3, 38, 70, 111
Coming out 79, 80, 133
   as political act 80
Community 15, 18, 81, 89, 105, 106, 126, 134, 144, 162, 164
Conformity 52, 53
Consciousness 17, 20, 79, 81, 108
   raising groups 78
Counselling 20, 23, 25, 27, 43, 50, 64, 78, 86, 143
Criminal/criminalization 20, 66
Culture
   cancel 82, 117
   offence 81
   wars 83

D
Defence/s 70, 147, 150, 151
Depression 42, 88
Diagnosis 31, 43, 54, 86
   psychiatric 88

Disruption 15, 38–41, 43
Dissonance 51, 60, 64, 67, 69
Drug/s 15–21, 90

E
Entitlement 42, 84
Environment 28, 31, 34, 59, 78, 86, 117, 129
Ethics 41, 63, 151, 161
Existential 14, 16, 22, 148, 153
   perspective 55
   phenomenology 62
Extinction Rebellion 82

F
Faith 32, 149, 152, 153
   bad 22, 53
Fear 15, 18, 23, 113, 126, 127, 131–134, 142, 155–157, 159
Fight 14, 18, 20, 98, 99, 126
Finitude 14, 19
Floyd, George 13, 39
Freedom 14, 22, 35, 41, 113, 130, 146, 148, 149, 152

G
Game of Thrones 77
Gaslight/gaslighting 39, 108, 118, 159
Gay 79–81, 116, 117, 120, 132, 134, 155, 156, 161
Gender 22, 39–41, 112, 125–127, 130, 132, 134
   trans 125, 132
Gift/s 28
Granger, Hermione 35

Grief 139, 140, 143

H
Hate 3, 17, 20, 51, 89, 97–100, 116–119
'Hearts and minds' 79, 83, 160
Heterosexual 80
Hilton, Paul 157
History Boys, The 52
HIV 3, 117, 121
Homelessness 14
Homophobia 1, 4, 41, 79, 117, 121, 128
  internalised 42
Horwood, Craig Revel 54
Humiliation 98, 100
Hunting 63, 66
  Act (2004) 64
  fox 63, 64, 66

I
Identification 152, 160
  with the aggressor 40
Immortality 14, 20
In/visibility 82, 161
Inequality 3, 22, 38, 86
Inheritance, The 157–160
Internalise 42, 109, 118, 126, 130, 132, 133
  homophobia 42
Interpretation 27, 59–62, 64, 66–69, 71–73, 152
Intersection/intersectionality 81, 82, 128
Isolation 22, 116, 149, 160

J
Junkyard 113
  room 104, 106, 113, 114
Justice 38, 82, 87, 98, 122, 134, 164

K
Khaleesi 77, 78

L
Language 16, 62, 82, 86, 110, 111, 117, 118, 134, 143
  English 109–111
Lewis, John 39
Liminal 14, 19
  state 14
Loss 18, 54, 112, 141, 144, 147, 157, 160
Love 1, 2, 20, 23, 51, 55, 63, 97, 98, 120–122, 139–142, 144, 146, 148, 161
Lunatic/s 17

M
Madame X 39, 40, 44
Madonna 39
McDonaldization 89
Meaning 15, 21, 22, 62, 64, 67, 71, 81, 90, 129, 132, 147, 149, 152, 153, 159
  lessness 55, 62, 119, 132
Mental health 4, 34, 42, 85, 86, 88
#MeToo 39
Microaggression 81, 108, 118
Misogynist 3, 42, 117
Misogyny 1, 4, 38, 118
Moffie 158, 160

Mormont, Jorah 77

N

Nature 1, 20, 22, 26–28, 34, 68, 86, 118, 121, 146, 152
Neoliberalism 158
New York 116, 160
NHS 34, 71, 88
Non-binary 117, 125–131, 134
Nothingness 14, 19, 21, 112

O

Objective/objectivity 4, 32, 49–51, 53, 55, 56, 87, 108, 149, 159
  objectivication 49–51, 53–57
  pseudo 55
Oppression 22, 41, 42, 78, 82, 86, 88, 112, 130
  historical 112
Othering 3, 130, 133
Other, The 2, 21, 22

P

Pathology 22, 43, 89
Politics/political 3–5, 20, 22, 23, 39, 40, 44, 57, 62, 63, 68, 72, 78–82, 85–90, 98, 119, 120, 143, 146, 147, 160
  party 79
Poverty 20, 22, 86
Power
  dynamics 28, 108, 109
  lessness 19, 40, 42, 43
  structure/s 42
Practice 3–5, 20, 26, 27, 29, 33, 41, 62, 82, 85, 87–89, 106, 119, 146, 151, 153, 161
  best 27, 56
  private 34
Precariousness 5, 6, 50, 159, 163
Prescription
  rights 90
Pride 81, 115, 150, 155
Prison 16, 20, 21
Projection 19, 79
Psychoanalysis 4, 40
Psychoanalytic 16, 29, 143
Psychologist/s 29, 30, 32, 60, 62, 68, 83, 87–90
  counselling 20, 23, 25, 64
  trainee 28
Psychology 2, 78, 83, 86, 88, 89, 163
  counselling 50, 78, 86
Psychotherapist/s 20, 23, 41–44, 87, 146

Q

Queer 116–119, 132, 160, 161

R

Race 70, 104, 107, 133, 147
Racism 22, 38, 39, 41, 107–109, 118, 128
Racist 3, 42, 107, 108, 110, 117, 128
Reasonable/reasonableness 39, 97
Reflective 4, 5, 25, 128, 139, 149
Rehabilitation 18
Relationality 163
Rules 14, 15, 26, 27, 29–31, 33–35, 38–41, 43, 52, 117, 127

S

Schitts Creek 160
Self
  deception 147, 151
  examination 129–131, 151
  harm 16
Sexism 22, 128
Shackleton, Sir Ernest 66–68
Shame 18–20, 80, 100, 106, 113, 120, 126, 133, 152, 156
Skunk Anansie 90
Slavery 108, 112
Smiths, The 68
Snowflake
  generation 82
Social
  justice 38, 82, 87, 134, 164
  justice agenda 87
  justice warrior 82
  media 39, 82
Socialisation 72
  primary 68
Soller, Kyle 157, 158
Splitting 3, 82, 89, 108
Status quo 38, 40–43, 52, 53
Stereotype/stereotyping 80
Storytelling 157–160, 162
Strictly Come Dancing 53, 54
Subject 18, 39, 42, 49, 53, 55, 71, 83, 86, 144, 147
  neo-liberal 83, 86
Subjectivity/subjectivities 53, 56, 83, 86, 88, 139, 147, 149
Suicide
  attempt 30
Supervision 28, 29, 31, 150, 151

T

Teaching 6, 57, 83, 98, 160
Tears 28, 101, 141, 153, 155, 158, 161
Thelma and Louise 119
Therapeutic 26–32, 34, 41, 42, 52, 88, 105, 106, 109, 149, 153
  process 150
Therapy 4, 6, 26, 28–34, 42, 43, 52, 57, 78, 87–90, 106, 107, 143, 150–152, 157, 159
The Seagull 145, 147
Thieves 17
Tonioli, Bruno 54
Transphobia 41, 118, 126, 128
Trauma/s 21, 42, 118, 142, 156, 161
  historic 112

U

Uncanny 5, 139, 142, 148, 150, 152, 159
Uncertainty 2, 17, 22, 146, 151
Unconscious 18, 19, 108, 110–112, 126

V

Van der Swart, Nicholas 160
Vegetarian 68, 71, 73
Violence
  interpersonal 18
  sexual 38
  systemic 18
Virtue
  signalling 82
Vulnerability 89, 103, 112, 113, 146–148, 153

W

War of the worlds, The 70
Wells, H.G. 70
Westminster
 Council 37, 39, 40

Witness 30, 82, 86, 99, 105, 143
Wizard of Oz 56

X

Xenophobia 22

The manufacturer's authorised representative in the EU is Springer Nature Customer Service Centre GmbH, Europaplatz 3, 69115 Heidelberg, Germany. If you have any concerns regarding our products, please contact ProductSafety@springernature.com

Printed and bound by CPI Group (UK) Ltd, Croydon, CR0 4YY

25/03/2026

02078205-0010